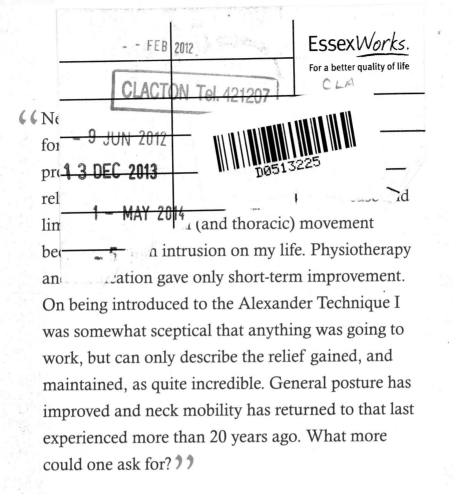

EssexWorks.
For a better quality of life
CLA

❝Ne
for
pr
rel   d
lin   (and thoracic) movement
be   n intrusion on my life. Physiotherapy
an   ation gave only short-term improvement.
On being introduced to the Alexander Technique I
was somewhat sceptical that anything was going to
work, but can only describe the relief gained, and
maintained, as quite incredible. General posture has
improved and neck mobility has returned to that last
experienced more than 20 years ago. What more
could one ask for?❞

Kieran Tobin, MB, B Ch, BAO, FRCS (Eng), FRCS (Irl), DLO;
Past-President of the Irish Otolaryngological, Head and Neck Society;
Past-President of the ENT Section of the Royal Society of Medicine of Ireland

Richard Brennan is an internationally renowned author, having written four books on the Alexander Technique, which have been translated into eight languages. He travels throughout Europe and the USA giving TV and radio interviews, running workshops and giving lectures. He is the co-founder of the Irish Society of Alexander Technique Teachers (ISATT) and lives in Galway, Ireland, where he runs a busy private practice as well as being the director of the Alexander Technique Teacher Training College, Ireland, which is recognized by the Society of Teachers of the Alexander Technique Teachers (STAT). **www.alexander.ie**

Other books by Richard Brennan
The Alexander Technique – Natural Poise for Health
The Alexander Technique Workbook
The Alexander Technique Manual
Mind and Body Stress Relief with the Alexander Technique
Stress – The Alternative Solution

CHANGE YOUR POSTURE
CHANGE YOUR LIFE

HOW THE POWER OF THE ALEXANDER TECHNIQUE CAN COMBAT BACK PAIN, TENSION AND STRESS

RICHARD BRENNAN

WATKINS PUBLISHING

LONDON

This edition first published in the UK and USA 2012 by
Watkins Publishing, Sixth Floor, Castle House,
75–76 Wells Street, London W1T 3QH

Design and typography copyright © Watkins Publishing 2012

1 3 5 7 9 10 8 6 4 2

Designed and typeset by Jerry Goldie Graphic Design

Printed and bound by Imago in China

British Library Cataloguing-in-Publication Data Available
Library of Congress Cataloging-in-Publication Data Available

ISBN: 978-1-78028-024-0

www.watkinspublishing.co.uk

Distributed in the USA and Canada by Sterling Publishing Co., Inc.
387 Park Avenue South, New York, NY 10016-8810

For information about custom editions, special sales, premium and corporate
purchases, please contact Sterling Special Sales Department at 800-805-5489 or
specialsales@sterlingpub.com

Contents

Introduction   1

Chapter 1   Alexander Technique – The Benefits   3

Chapter 2   The Origin of the Technique   19

Chapter 3   The Development of the Technique   29

Chapter 4   How the Alexander Technique Works   36

Chapter 5   Understanding Posture   53

Chapter 6   Posture and Education   64

Chapter 7   The Secret Key to Good Posture   76

Chapter 8   The Effects of Furniture on Posture   85

Chapter 9   The Hidden Obstacle to Improving Posture   100

Chapter 10   Your Inner Acrobat   115

Chapter 11   Inside Yourself   131

Chapter 12   Posture and Shoes   138

Chapter 13   First Steps to Improving Posture   147

Chapter 14   Posture and Breathing   157

Chapter 15   Bringing Your Life Back Into Balance   168

Appendix   Randomized controlled trial of Alexander Technique lessons, exercise and massage (ATEAM) for chronic and recurrent back pain   177

Understanding the Terminology   179

Resources   180

Further Reading   182

Index   183

Acknowledgments

I would like to thank the following long list of people who have supported me in the writing of this book. First, I would like to give very special thanks to my wife, Caroline, for the initial proof reading and making suggestions about improvements, a great deal of computer support as well as helping with the photo-shoot. Secondly, I am very grateful to Dr Miriam Wohl, a friend, Alexander teacher and a medically trained doctor who gave generously of her time and of herself for a second (and third!) proof reading and for the many interesting discussions we had along the way. I would like to thank Kieran Tobin for writing his wonderful endorsement of the Technique at the beginning of the book and I would also like to thank the following teachers who have helped in many different ways with the production of the book: Giora Pinkas, Jessica Wolfe, Glenna Batson and Ingrid Bacci. Also I would like to say a big thank you to all those involved in the photo-shoot: the photographer, Brad Anderson, and the models, Ciaran Brennan, Laoise Brennan and Michaela Wohlgemuth, and to Julia Brown for her much needed help with the illustrations and to Paul Cook and Jeremy Chance with their help in finding the photographs of F Matthias Alexander and Jean Fisher for permission to print an extract from, The Philosophers Stone. Thanks also to my agent, Susan Mears, for initiating the project and my editor Alison Bolus for all her hard work. Lastly, but not least, I would like to thank all those people working behind the scenes at Watkins Publishing, including Michael Mann, Penny Stopa and Jerry Goldie in the production and distribution of this book.

For Cara, Tim, Ciaran and Laoise

Introduction

Are you tired of the effects of poor posture in your life? Do you feel frustrated that anything you do to try to improve your posture doesn't seem to work? Would you like a relaxed, yet upright posture, beautiful balance and graceful coordination? If so, then this book is for you!

In this book I hope to convey a simple message: your posture directly affects your body's overall functioning and has a major influence on how you think and feel. Poor posture can also adversely affect the position and functioning of your vital organs and cause more health problems than you realize. Many people with chronic pain can trace their problems to years of faulty postural habits.

Good posture, by contrast, promotes free movement and physical and mental endurance, improves appearance and contributes to an overall feeling of wellbeing. Good posture allows the body's healing processes to work more efficiently and effectively, and helps to prevent future illness. Good posture aligns your body and helps your muscles, joints and ligaments to do their job as nature intended. Improving posture reduces fatigue, muscular strain and pain. Good posture brings the body back into balance, physically, mentally and emotionally. A person who has good, natural posture tends to project poise, confidence, integrity and dignity.

This book is emphatically *not* about sitting up straight, pulling your shoulders back and arching your back, as you may often have been told to do in the past. It is about finding your natural poise again: that wonderful, graceful posture that you naturally had as a child. You will find that if you improve your posture, you will improve the quality of your life. Although the main theme of this book is to explain what the Alexander Technique is and how it can be used to improve posture, I will also explore the effects of external factors, such as chairs and shoes, on posture. I need to make it clear, however, that although these are nothing to do with the Technique as such, I have personally found that these can also be very helpful in my life and when teaching others.

Before we start exploring ways of improving posture, let me first explain how this book came about. Over the last 20 years I have run hundreds of Alexander Technique classes and workshops, and the number of people who have attended must be over 10,000 by now. One of the first things I ask the participants is: 'How many of you would like to improve your posture?' Every time, without fail, nearly everyone puts their hand up without a moment's hesitation. The reasons given for wanting to improve posture vary greatly. Some people suffer from various muscular complaints, such as hip, back or neck problems, while others have asthma, stress or various types of Repetitive Strain Injury (RSI). Quite a few may have no physical pain at all, but just want to look better and improve their general coordination and ease of movement. Some simply want to improve their self-esteem. Whatever the reason, however, it seems that many, many people are aware that 'bad posture' is a large part of their problem.

I wasn't really surprised that some people in the class wanted to improve their posture, after all, it is well known that the Alexander Technique can be very beneficial in this area; what surprised me though was that in *every* class, practically *everyone* felt that they had poor posture and *everyone* wanted to improve it! In fact, in a recent survey conducted by a leading glamour magazine, women were asked if they were happy with their general posture. Out of the thousands of women who were questioned, not one woman said that she was happy with it. After a while it dawned on me – practically everyone wants to improve something about their posture, but hardly anyone knows how to go about it in a way that is effective and long-lasting.

The other thing that I found very interesting was that although many people knew that muscular tension was causing or exacerbating their poor posture, they were still trying to improve it by tensing up even further. So for example, I saw people attempting to sit or stand up 'straight', but actually over-arching their backs in the attempt, or trying to 'pull their shoulders back' but in fact over-tensing their shoulders and upper back muscles. If you look at the natural and beautiful posture of a young child, it is evident that they are often very upright, but they are not *doing anything* to be upright. It is their natural way of being and they do not have to use any extra muscular effort to obtain such beautiful posture. It is just *there* because of their inbuilt postural reflexes doing the job for them without any conscious effort on their part – it is their birthright, and it is ours too.

I sincerely hope that you enjoy the book and find it helpful, not only in improving your posture but also in helping you to lead a more fulfilling and conscious life.

CHAPTER 1

Alexander Technique – the Benefits

After one Alexander session it felt like someone had poured a full canister of oil into my neck. After two sessions, I felt 20 years of neck tension fade away and I felt my chest naturally expand. I used to wrap myself round my instrument for years and when your head is inside the music, it's like an anesthetic, you don't feel the discomfort but the technique helped me to become aware of how I had been causing myself problems.

Máirtín O'Connor Traditional Irish Accordion player

For many people, the Alexander Technique is synonymous with improving posture, yet few are aware of exactly, how it works, and even Alexander Technique teachers themselves use differing language and emphasis in their explanation of it. It can sometimes come across as a purely physical technique, whereby we examine the way we sit, stand or move while learning to release muscular tension. At other times the emphasis can be looking at how our mental habits are reflected in the body, and by changing our thinking we change our posture. Yet for me, while it is both of these, it is also a practical philosophy for living, a way of becoming a more conscious human being, a way of finding our true potential. In fact, the Technique can be many different things to different people. All are correct, for these are just facets of the same thing.

Practical experience

What most people would agree upon, however, is that the Alexander Technique imparts an experience – a truly wonderful experience. But how you convey this amazing feeling into words is one of the most difficult problems. How do you convey the taste of a mango or pear to someone who has never tasted that fruit before? It is impossible. My first contact with the Alexander Technique in 1984, when I met my first teacher, Danny Reilly, is a very good example of this. We sat and talked by an open fire for nearly an hour about the subject of the Alexander Technique in great detail, but at the end of the conversation I just thought: 'What is this man talking about?' Then he said, 'I will show you in a practical way if you like.' Within a few minutes of having the hands-on experience, I began to have a profound experience of expanding gently in space. At the end of half an hour, I felt very light, free and very conscious of the world around me, but I no longer felt like me! The postural habits that I had associated with who I was had been removed. It was a moment that I remember to this day.

The famous actor and comedian John Cleese also found Alexander lessons very useful, reporting: 'I find the Alexander Technique very helpful in my work. Things happen without you trying. They get to be light and relaxed. You must get an Alexander teacher to show it to you.' Similarly, the author of very many well-known children's books, Roald Dahl, said, 'The Alexander Technique really works. I recommend it enthusiastically to anyone who has neck pains or back pain. I speak from experience.' But these statements cannot give you the experience; they can only encourage you to learn more and perhaps seek out a teacher who can show you how you can have a first-hand experience of lightness, wholeness and wellbeing.

I have found over the years that the reason why the Alexander Technique is difficult to describe is because it has a chameleon-like nature: the Technique can appear to change depending on the nature of the problem and how one approaches it. For this reason, it would probably be useful first to map out the areas in which the Alexander Technique can be beneficial, before we explain how it works. I have personally found that the Alexander Technique has greatly helped people in the following areas:

- Alleviating pain

- Improving posture

- Preserving health

- Reducing stress

- Enhancing performance

- Helping with personal development

- Increasing enjoyment of the present

Alleviating pain

This is perhaps the most common reason why people learn the Technique in the first place, as it is well known for helping people who are in pain or discomfort for a wide variety of reasons. Like me (I originally suffered with major back problems and sciatica), many people have sought help elsewhere without success; the Alexander Technique is often the last resort. In many cases pain is simply the body's alarm system, it is just saying 'Stop doing this to me', but the only problem is that we do not know what we are doing to ourselves, and as a consequence we have no idea that there is anything to stop. Marjorie Barlow, Alexander's niece and one of the first Alexander teachers, put it very simply when she said that the Technique enables you to know what you are doing and empowers you to stop doing whatever it is you are doing at any time you like.

The initial question we need to ask is: how can we identify the harmful things we are doing to ourselves? This is a very difficult thing to do without help, and an Alexander teacher has been trained to notice the harmful habits that we cannot see for ourselves. So, for example, I have seen many people with lower back pain over-arching their backs, thinking that this is improving their posture and will eventually fix their problem. Quite the opposite is true, however, and this tendency of 'sitting up straight' can actually make it worse and may even have caused the pain in the first place. Similarly, I've

1: The way we stand or sit can often put unnecessary strain on our body without us realizing it.

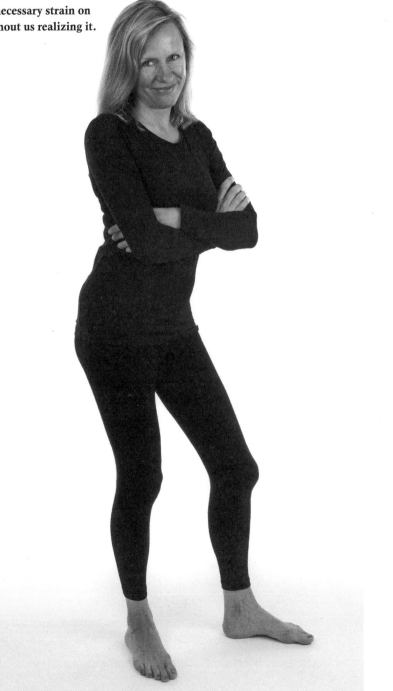

seen people with neck problems throwing their heads back with a great deal of force when getting out of a chair, but have no idea that they are doing so. I also come across a lot of people with numerous musculoskeletal problems who think they are standing straight but are actually leaning backwards at a 10 or 15 degree angle, and I've seen others who suffer from frequent headaches and migraine, but are totally unaware that they are continually over-tensing their neck muscles. With so much tension around, it is little wonder that so many millions experience lower back pain or neck problems. I can honestly say that if we did to others what we do to ourselves, we could be arrested for grievous bodily harm! Yet many of us don't know the harm we are causing ourselves.

Some people say that the trouble with the human body is that it does not come with a 'user manual'. Life might be much simpler if it did. However, young children don't have a user manual, but they generally move, sit and stand with beautiful poise and balance. Actually, we don't need a manual – all we need to do is to let go of the unconscious habits that cause so many of the physical problems that we see in society today. A good analogy of this was reported in a newspaper some years ago. An American woman arrived at Heathrow Airport in London from New York. She rented a car because she wanted to visit relatives in Scotland, and proceeded up the M1 motorway. When she got to Edinburgh, she took the car back to the car rental company and complained bitterly that there was something wrong with the car. She reported that the engine was very noisy and the car was very slow, and that it had taken her twice as long as expected to get to Scotland. A mechanic checked the car and could find nothing wrong with it. The woman was dismayed and she tried to show the mechanic what was wrong. At that point it became evident that she had never driven a car with gears – she had always driven a car with an automatic gearbox. So she had put the car into first gear and didn't realize that she needed to change gears when picking up speed! Of course the car was very noisy and didn't go very fast! So, there was no problem with the car – the fact was that the driver was not driving the car as it had been designed to be driven. In exactly the same way we do not 'drive' ourselves in the way that we were designed to be driven; most of us misuse ourselves for many years before a variety of health problems arise. The power of the Alexander Technique is in revealing this misuse and allowing a person to restore their health for themselves.

A person can learn to change harmful habits once they have this new awareness.

In this book, I aim to go some of the way towards helping you to understand how the body is designed to work, so that with the help of the Alexander Technique you will be able to use yourself with more consideration and awareness and thus move through life with greater ease and less pain or discomfort.

Improving posture

In my experience, the second most common reason people come to me is to improve their posture, either because people around them have commented on it or because they themselves have caught sight of their posture in a mirror. They want better deportment, and wish to learn how to sit, stand and move more gracefully and attractively. Poor posture is rife in our society today, and it is rare to meet someone who does not want to improve their posture in some way. I remember seeing a *Peanuts* cartoon a long time ago that resonated with me. In the cartoon, Peppermint Patty, who is standing very upright, is speaking to Marcie. She says, 'What kind of a report card is this? I got a D minus for everything! Look at my back, Marcie. It's straight isn't it? Doesn't good posture count for anything?!' That is a very good question! The answer is yes, it counts for a great deal in this life.

Although Alexander did on occasion use the word 'posture' in his writing, he did not like the word because he felt that it implied something static rather than dynamic, and thought that it might encourage habits rather than freedom. Instead, he more usually referred to '*the use of the self*' or '*the way we use ourselves*', of which posture was the physical expression of something far bigger than just the shape of the body. Throughout the book we will see that we cannot successfully alter our posture without regard for the way we think and feel. So I wish to make it quite clear that when I use the word 'posture', I do so in a wider sense that encompasses our whole being: body, mind, spirit and emotions.

The idea that posture affects health, wellbeing and happiness is an ancient one; many different disciplines have studied, defined and described health-related benefits to posture throughout the ages. Good posture has been depicted in the artwork of ancient civilizations and presented in the practice

2: Even though our bodies are under strain in certain positions, that way of sitting eventually becomes habitual and after a time may even 'feel' comfortable to us.

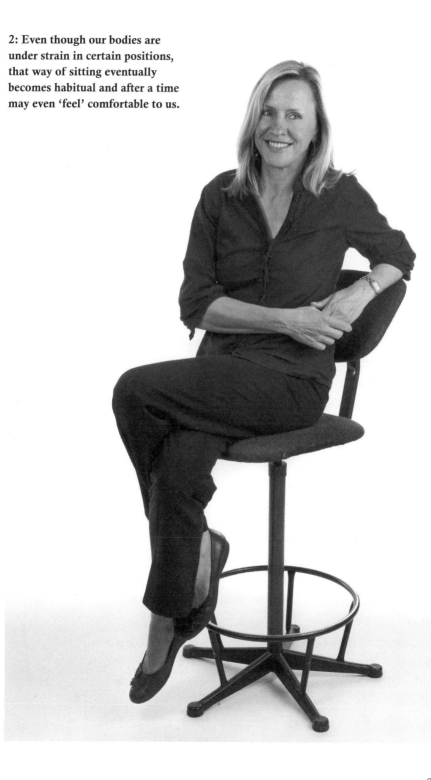

of yoga and the martial arts – disciplines that have been taught down through the ages. Much has been told of posture and its relationship to health and longevity, dating back thousands of years to the ancient Greeks, Romans and Egyptians. But today, the idea that postural characteristics can be a direct cause of poor health is virtually disregarded in the clinical practice of many physicians. Before improving posture, however, we first need to understand how the postural reflexes work; this will be covered in the next chapter.

Preserving health

By learning the Alexander Technique, you can maintain good health into your old age. There are three examples that I'd like to share with you. The first is of a friend and colleague, Elisabeth Walker. She trained with F M Alexander and became an Alexander teacher in 1947. I first met her in 2000 at an Alexander Technique conference, when she was in her mid-eighties, still travelling the world to give workshops and inspire people. Four years later, at another Alexander Congress, she was seen frequently riding her bike around Oxford at the age of 90. At the same Congress, she took part in a workshop that involved walking on a tightrope. Even today, in her mid-nineties, she is still actively teaching and travelling.

The second example is of a woman who came to me when she was 96. She had had Alexander lessons since the age of 30, and many of her first lessons were with Alexander himself. She was still driving and attending a

❝ Mr Alexander has done a service to the subject by insistently treating each act as involving the whole integrated individual, the whole psycho-physical man. To take a step is an affair not of this or that limb solely, but of the total neuromuscular activity of the moment – not the least of the head and neck. ❞

Sir Charles Sherrington, Nobel Prize winner in Physiology or Medicine, 1932

number of evening classes. Every year she had some lessons from different Alexander teachers, 'just to keep her hand in', as she put it. After her first lesson with me, she said, 'I would like another one, but not next week as I am going on a skiing holiday.' This woman was still skiing at the age of 96!

The third example I would like to give is of George Bernard Shaw. He was 80 and suffering with acute pain due to angina and then over-curvature of the lumbar spine when he arrived for his first lesson with Alexander. It affected him so badly that he could hardly take a step without agony; in fact, he was so frail that he needed help to get up the three steps to Alexander's teaching rooms. It really seemed that he was on his last legs. Shaw believed that his angina was a direct consequence of sitting for long periods and hunching over his writing desk. He thought that this habit had put enormous pressure onto his heart so it could not work efficiently, and during his lessons he was able to release the tension and give his heart room to function properly. Shaw proved to be the quickest to learn the Technique of all of Alexander's pupils. In less than three weeks the pain had eased and he was able to walk a mile as well as resume his daily swimming routine. After a course of lessons, he proclaimed himself 'a new man' and went on to live another 14 years in excellent health and didn't die until the age of 94, after he fell off a ladder while pruning his trees. Now if you think about it, you don't get many 94-year-olds up ladders in the first place, especially when 14 years before they were unable to get up three steps. In private, he gave Alexander the credit for saving his life, and he advised Alexander to hire a man to walk up and down Piccadilly in London carrying a sandwich board that said 'ALEXANDER CURES ANGINA' on both sides. He was sure that it would have made Alexander a public success overnight.

After his course of lessons, Shaw is reported to have said to Alexander, 'I am very grateful to you for restoring me to good health. My angina and back problem are completely cured and I feel like I am moving like a young man again. However, you have left me with one problem that I did not have before; now that I'm three inches taller and two inches wider in the shoulders – none of my suits fit me anymore.' All through his eighties and early nineties he was known to be 'very sprightly', and he continued to lead a very full and active life. In public he declared: 'Alexander established not only the beginnings of a far reaching science of the apparently involuntary movements we call reflexes, but a technique of correction and self-control which forms a substantial addition to our very slender resources in personal education.'

Reducing stress

There are differing opinions in the medical profession as to whether prolonged stress can be a direct cause of illness. Some doctors believe that stress can cause high blood pressure and an increase in the level of harmful fats in the blood, which is a contributory cause of heart disease and hypertension. Others believe that excessive tension over a period of time causes a reduction in the body's own defence mechanisms, and as a result people under stress are more prone to a wide range of diseases because their resistance has been weakened. Whichever way you look at it, stress is bad for your health, and it may even lead to premature death through strokes or heart disease, or by accidents caused by impaired judgement or performance.

Let's take the example of the habitual reaction that typically arises when we are running late for an appointment. Many of us respond by tensing the whole body, hunching our shoulders, clenching our teeth or arching our back. As we fear the consequences of being late, we are no longer in conscious control of our actions and may well act irrationally. If we are driving, we may even take unnecessary risks that could threaten our own or other people's lives. This in turn can make us even more stressed, and a vicious circle ensues. This kind of habitual reaction eventually becomes so ingrained that we maintain excessive muscle tension even when we think we are relaxed.

The fearful responses we experience often originate during our school years, when being late often resulted in some form of ridicule or punishment, and, like Pavlov's dogs, we still respond in a similar fashion many years later, even when being late for an appointment is of little importance. If this behaviour pattern is allowed to persist over a long period of time, we may end up suffering from one of the many stress-related illnesses. When we are stressed, our posture changes dramatically, and that change may become permanent if we are stressed frequently (as happens all too often). The Alexander Technique can help us to become aware of our current stress levels, as well as helping us to become less stressed.

Enhancing performance

In fact, the Technique can help you to improve whatever you do. Alexander was once reported to say that even a thief practising his Technique would become a better thief!

There are three main areas where the Technique can improve performance:

- Sport

- Music

- Acting and public speaking

Sport

The Alexander Technique has been known to help all kinds of sportsmen and women throughout the world, both at amateur levels and in training for high-pressure competitions. Since the way you use your body can affect your performance, it follows that the more aware you are of your actions, the greater the control you will have of your body. The Alexander Technique has been used effectively in a wide variety of different sports, from swimming to athletics (many professional runners are always looking for new styles of running that are not only more efficient, but also less strenuous). It is also very well known in horse-riding circles because the rider's posture clearly affects the performance of the horse.

Many sports place huge demands on the body and can lead to injury in the form of twisted ankles, torn ligaments and sometimes even broken bones. Using the Technique to reduce tension in demanding activities can dramatically lessen the risk of injury as well as increase freedom and flexibility. Not only does this help to bring about improvements in performance, but many people also find that their sport becomes more enjoyable. Many forms of training invite the sportsperson to try harder and harder, which can result in extra tension in an already strained muscular system. This can put enormous pressures on the body, and if allowed to persist can interfere with its natural mechanisms and be counter productive. Sometimes, due to pain caused by excessive tension, sportspeople even have to give up their favourite sport altogether. But if and when they are able to give up their old habitual ways of straining, they can be amazed to find that an easier, more flowing style can produce the same, or even better, results – with less effort. Equestrian Sally

13

Swift, author of *Centred Riding*, used the principles of the Alexander Technique in her teaching and aptly described it as a method of re-educating the mind and body towards greater balance and integration, with special reference to posture and movement.

In all forms of sport, improving posture and the use of the whole self can help to improve general fitness and teach you how to avoid wasting energy. It can also help you to avoid or recover more quickly from an injury. Greg Chappell, the well-known Australian test cricketer, said: 'The Alexander Technique will benefit anyone whether they are an elite athlete or whether they just wish to live life without the aches and pains that many people suffer and accept as part of life. It is a pity that these techniques are not shown to us all at an early age for I have no doubt that this would alleviate many of the causes of ill health in our communities.' For his part, Howard Payne, Commonwealth record hammer thrower, who used the Technique to improve his balance, said: 'Balance is a vital aspect of good hammer throwing and getting the head, neck, spine and pelvis in the correct relationship enables the balance of the throw to come so much more easily. Once the balance is settled there is an enormous improvement in turning speed.'

Many sportsmen and women have used the Technique in improving performance. Daley Thompson won four world records, two Olympic gold medals and three Commonwealth titles and had wins in the World and European Championships. He is considered by many to be the greatest decathlete of all time. Other sportspeople who have found the Technique useful include John McEnroe (tennis), Linford Christie (sprinter) and Jeff Julian (golf).

Music

Musicians all over the world use the Technique to improve their performance. The Alexander Technique has helped many instrumentalists and singers to perform with less stress, more confidence and a reduction in pain or injury. At performance level, many musicians and singers are required to undertake very demanding physical movements. These movements often cause back problems, neck problems, Repetitive Strain Injury (RSI) – a term used to describe an injury of the musculoskeletal and nervous systems that may be caused by repetitive tasks, forceful exertions, vibrations, mechanical compression or sustained or awkward positions – and a wide range of

3: Children often have a natural ease about them, no matter what they are doing.

4: In contrast to children, adults are inclined to apply excessive muscular tension while performing a variety of tasks. Compare the position of the shoulders between this man and the child, who are both involved in the same activity.

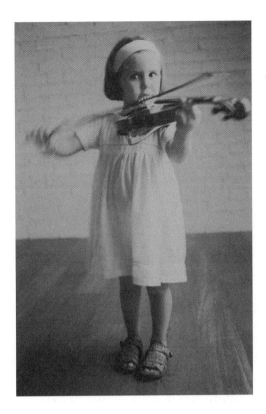

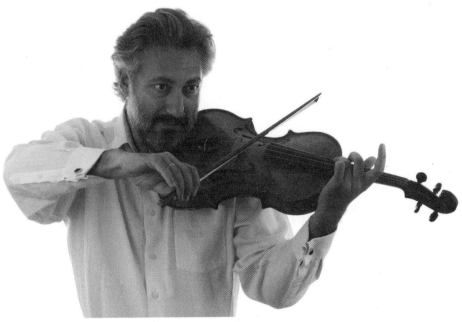

undiagnosed health problems that can adversely affect or even threaten their musical career. By helping musicians to improve the way they use themselves while playing any musical instrument or while singing, performers have less risk of injury, and this improves the quality of the music itself.

Improving posture with the Alexander Technique can also dramatically reduce performance nerves and increase the performer's confidence in a variety of situations. Many of the major acting and music schools, such as Royal College of Music (London), The Royal Conservatory of Music (Toronto), DIT Conservatory of Music and Drama (Dublin), The Yehudi Menuhin School (Cobham, UK), Royal Academy of Dramatic Art (RADA) (London) and The Juilliard School (New York), regularly have Alexander teachers working with the students to help them become more aware of what they are doing.

Over the years, a great number of prominent musicians and actors have publicly endorsed the Alexander Technique, and their comments on the efficacy of the Technique can be found throughout the book.

Acting and public speaking

It was from the field of acting that the Alexander Technique originated. The Technique can offer many benefits in the world of acting and public speaking. By improving the way performers use themselves, their voices will naturally be clearer and more powerful without being forced. Actors can also learn to perceive the habits that get in the way of obtaining their best

❝ Mr Alexander's method lays hold of the individual as a whole, as a self-vitalizing agent. He reconditions and re-educates the reflex mechanisms and brings their habits into normal relation with the functioning of the organism as a whole. I regard this method as thoroughly scientific and educationally sound. ❞

Professor George E Coghill, anatomist and physiologist, member of
National Academy of Sciences

performance. These habits can include patterns of thought and physical misperceptions that encourage actors and public speakers to use excessive and unnecessary tension and effort. Professional performers can learn to free their breath, which helps them to express strong emotions on stage with effortless poise, and move with grace and ease on and off the stage.

Helping with personal development

The Technique can enable a person to be more aware physically, mentally and emotionally in a variety of situations. A large part of learning the Technique involves learning how we behave in certain situations, and how we react to a wide range of stimuli; but being more conscious of how we go about our daily activities can teach us a lot about ourselves. As we become aware of our personal reactions, we are slowly able to change them for the better. The expression by Mark Twain, 'If you do what you always did, you will get what you always got.' is so true. The Technique has been referred to by some as a quiet revolution in self-development. As we will see, the mind, the emotions and the body are intrinsically one entity. It is not just that each affects the other; it is that they are all different facets of the same thing. Alter the body and you will alter the way you think and feel, and vice versa. By learning the Alexander Technique you will be embarking on a journey of self-discovery. You will discover things that will amaze and delight you. It is a humbling experience and one of the first things to realize is how little we really know, despite having more education than ever before. It is not a journey to be rushed, so take your time and savour the process.

Increasing enjoyment of the present

There are many inspiring books about the benefits of living in the present, such as *The Power of Now* by Eckhart Tolle, and *Awareness* by Anthony de Mello. By practising the Alexander Technique, you will find a practical way to be really present in this world. Our mind can disappear into the past or shoot off into the future at a moment's notice, and emotions are always moving like the tides of the oceans, but in reality we are always here and now. When we are able to be present with the mindfulness that is the core of practising the Technique, we are able let go of the past and stop worrying about the future and truly be in the present moment. The present moment contains the magic and wonder that children see and feel every day.

Many people come to me with back pain, neck problems, hip problems, breathing problems and a whole range of other ailments. Once they have started using the Technique, even before their problems have been solved, they start to report that they are sleeping better, feel happier and are more present. In the last years of Alexander's life, he once said to his niece, Marjorie Barlow, 'You know something? I am always happy.' Happiness is the thing that so many of us are chasing but that often becomes more and more elusive as we get older. You can see happiness in people's posture, and you can also see depression and sadness and unhappiness in their posture too. Change the posture by changing the way you use yourself, and you change the state of mind; change the way you think, and you change your life.

CHAPTER 2

The Origin of the Technique

This story of perceptiveness, of intelligence, and of persistence shown by a man without any medical training, is one of the true epics of medical research and practice.

Professor Nikolaas Tinbergen, Nobel Prize winner in Physiology or Medicine

The story of Frederick Matthias Alexander is a truly remarkable one by any standards. He was born in Australia on 20 January 1869, the eldest of the eight children of John and Betsy Alexander. He was of mixed Scottish and Irish descent. He grew up near the small town of Wynyard, situated on the north-west coast of the island of Tasmania. So our story starts at a time when there was no electricity, no telephones and no computers. Horses and walking were the main forms of transport, and self-sufficiency was a way of life.

The early years

Alexander was born prematurely, and from the start he was a very sickly child, suffering from respiratory problems. Due to his frail health, he was taken out of school at an early age and tutored in the evenings by the local schoolteacher. Even as a young boy he was very inquisitive and was in some ways difficult to teach, and he used to ask his teacher how he could be certain that the information he was being taught was correct. During the day he helped his father look after horses, and I am sure that the sensitivity in his hands that was later to play such a crucial part in his teaching of the Technique to others was partly due to that.

As he got older, Alexander's health gradually improved, and by the time he was 17, financial pressures within the family had forced him to leave the outdoor life of which he had become so fond, to work in the Mount Bischoff Tin Mining Company. During this time he taught himself to play the violin and took part in some amateur dramatics. At the age of 20 he had saved £500 (a small fortune in those days) and travelled to Melbourne, where he stayed with his uncle, James Pearce, and passed the next three months spending his hard-earned savings on going to the theatre and concerts and visiting art galleries. At the end of this period, Alexander had firmly decided to train to be an actor and reciter.

The young actor

Alexander stayed on in Melbourne and took on various jobs, working for an estate agent, in a department store and even as a tea-taster for a tea merchant to finance his training, which he did in the evenings and at weekends. It was not long before he gained a fine reputation as a first-class reciter, and he went on to form his own theatre company specializing in one-man Shakespeare recitals. As he became increasingly successful, Alexander began to accept more and more engagements, his audiences got bigger, and consequently so did the halls in which he performed. With no microphones, this put more and more strain on his voice. After a while, the strain began to show, as he regularly became hoarse in the middle of his performances. He approached a variety of people, including doctors and voice trainers, who gave him medication and exercises, but nothing seemed to make any difference. In fact, the situation deteriorated still further, until on one occasion Alexander could barely finish his recital.

He became more and more anxious as he realized that his entire career was in jeopardy. Increasingly desperate, he approached his doctor again, even though previous treatment had not worked. After a fresh examination of Alexander's throat, the doctor was convinced that the vocal cords had merely been overstrained and prescribed complete rest of his voice for two weeks, promising that this would give Alexander a solution to his problem. Determined to try anything, Alexander used his voice as little as possible for the two-week period preceding his next important engagement. He found that the hoarseness in his voice slowly disappeared.

At the beginning of the performance, Alexander was delighted to find that his voice was crystal clear; in fact, it was better than it had been for a long time. His delight soon turned into huge disappointment, however, when halfway through his performance the hoarseness returned and the condition continued to deteriorate until by the end of the evening he could hardly speak.

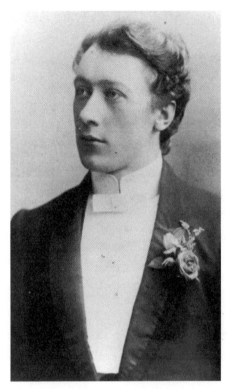

Frederick Matthias Alexander

The next day he returned to his doctor to report what had happened. The doctor felt that his recommendation had had some effect and advised him to continue with the treatment. What transpired next proved to be at the very heart of the Alexander Technique.

Early experiments

Alexander refused any further treatment, arguing that after two weeks of following the doctor's instructions implicitly, his problem had returned within an hour. He reasoned with the doctor that if his voice was perfect when he started the recital, and yet was in a terrible state by the time he had finished, *it must have been something that he was doing while performing that was causing the problem.* The doctor thought carefully and agreed that this must be the case. 'Can you tell me, then, what it was that caused the trouble?' Alexander asked. The doctor honestly admitted that he could not. To which Alexander replied,

'Very well. If that is so, I must try and find out for myself.'

Alexander left the surgery very determined to find a solution to his curious problem. This took him on a journey of discovery that not only gave him the answer to his question, but also ultimately led to a profound new understanding of how human beings are designed to move and how the body and mind and the emotions are inseparable. He came to realize that many people grossly interfere with their own natural movement and that this contributes to much of mankind's suffering in our modern civilization. Alexander's findings were greatly underestimated at the time, but it can be argued that his discovery was one of the greatest of the 20th century.

You may now be thinking that you have no problem with your own voice – perhaps you have a different problem, so how can the Technique help you? Alexander's logic can be applied to practically any ailment we have. For example, if someone has no back pain before they do the gardening, yet has back pain after doing the gardening, then it must follow that they are putting their body under undue stress while digging or weeding and that this is the underlying cause of the problem. It does not matter what physical ailment you are suffering from, and what activity might bring it on; there is always an underlying cause, and when that is addressed, the pain or discomfort will gradually disappear.

The first clues

As you will see, Alexander's story is like a Sherlock Holmes mystery. Alexander's genius was his insight that he could be causing his own problems himself without realizing it. Through his tenacity he came to prove it, and to cure himself. How many people do you know with back or neck problems who have ever had the thought that they may be causing the problem themselves? Alexander had only two clues to follow up when he started his investigations:

1. The act of reciting on stage brought about the hoarseness that caused him to lose his voice.

2. When speaking in a normal manner, the hoarseness in his voice disappeared.

Following simple, logical steps, Alexander deduced that if ordinary speaking did not cause him to lose his voice, while reciting did, there must be something different about what he did while speaking normally and what he did when reciting. If he could find out what that difference was, he might be able to change the way in which he was using his voice when reciting, which would then solve his problem. He used a mirror to observe himself both when speaking in his normal voice and again when reciting, in the hope that he could discern some differences between the two. He watched carefully, but could see nothing wrong or unnatural while speaking normally. It was when he began to recite that he noticed several actions that were different:

1. He tended to pull his head back and down onto his spine with a certain amount of force.

2. He simultaneously depressed his larynx (the cavity in the throat where the vocal cords are situated).

3. He also began to suck air in through his mouth, which produced a gasping sound.

Up until this point, Alexander had been completely unaware of these habits, and when he returned to his normal speaking voice he realized that the same tendencies were also present but to a lesser extent, which was why they had previously gone undetected. So Alexander's first discovery was:

Interference with the physiological mechanisms often occurs habitually and unconsciously.

After this breakthrough, he returned to the mirror with new enthusiasm and recited over and over again to see if he could find any more clues, and soon noticed that the three tendencies became accentuated when he was reading passages in which unusual demands were made on his voice. This confirmed his earlier suspicion that there was a causal link between the way in which he recited and the strain on his voice.

A maze of questions

The next stumbling block that Alexander encountered was that he was unsure of the root cause of these damaging tendencies. He found himself lost in a maze of questions:

1. Was it the sucking in of the air while breathing that caused the pulling back of the head and the depressing of the larynx?

   or

2. Was it the pulling back of the head that caused the depressing of the larynx and the sucking in of the air?

   or

3. Was it the depressing of the larynx that caused the sucking in of the air and the pulling back of the head?

After further experimentation, he realized that he could not directly prevent the sucking in of the air while breathing or the depression of the larynx, but he could to some extent prevent the pulling back of the head by releasing muscular tension. When he did this he also noticed that it indirectly improved the state of the larynx and the breathing. At this point Alexander wrote in his journal: '*The importance of this discovery cannot be over-estimated, for through it I was led on to the further discovery of the primary control of the working of all the mechanisms of the human organism, and this marked the first important stage of my investigation.*'

Alexander's second discovery was:

> **The existence of the Primary Control, which organizes balance and coordination throughout the rest of the body.**

Alexander referred to the dynamic relationship between the head, neck and back as the 'Primary Control' and discovered that it governed the workings of all the body's mechanisms and made the control of the complex human being relatively simple. Freedom of movement requires the Primary Control to be allowed to work without any restriction so that the head can lead a movement and the rest of the body follows.

Alexander carried on with his experiments and soon found that when he prevented himself from pulling his head back and down onto his spine the hoarseness in his voice decreased. He returned to his doctor and after further examination it was found that there had been a considerable improvement in the general condition of his throat and vocal cords. He now had positive proof that the manner in which he was reciting was causing him to lose his voice, and he was encouraged to think that changing the way in which he performed would eventually lead to an eradication of his problem. Alexander's third discovery was:

The way in which a person uses themselve will invariably affect their various functions.

Unreliable sensory appreciation

Encouraged with the idea that he was at last getting to the heart of the matter, Alexander continued experimenting to see if he could achieve further improvement in the state of his vocal cords. He had observed a tendency to pull his head back, so in an attempt to correct this, he deliberately put his head forward. However, he was very surprised to find that this depressed the larynx just as much. To help him unravel this mystery, he added two further mirrors, one on each side of the original one. When he observed himself again in the mirrors, he could see clearly that he was still pulling his head back and down onto his spine as before, despite his intentions. Alexander realized that he was doing the exact opposite of what he thought he was doing. He had just made his next discovery:

The existence of faulty sensory appreciation

In other words, he could no longer rely on his sensory feeling alone to tell him accurately what he was or was not doing. At first he thought that this was his own personal idiosyncrasy, but later on, when he started to teach his technique to others, he realized that faulty sensory appreciation was practically universal. Feeling disillusioned, yet unable to give up his quest, Alexander persevered and began to notice that his habit of pulling his head back and down was causing not only the depression of his larynx but also various tensions and stresses throughout his entire body. He saw that he was also lifting his chest, arching his back, throwing his pelvis forward, over-tightening his leg muscles and even gripping the floor with his feet. The way he was holding his head was affecting his entire posture and balance. Alexander's next realization was:

The body does not function as a collection of separate independent parts, but as a whole unit, with every part affecting every other part.

———•———

Alexander remembered that during his training he had been taught to 'take hold of the floor' with his feet by one of his recital tutors. He had obeyed by tensing his feet and toes, believing that his teacher obviously knew better than he did. Many of us will remember being told to sit or stand in a certain way in order to correct poor posture. Even if we achieve what we think is being asked of us, in reality we may well make the situation worse instead of better. We are under the illusion that other people know what good posture is, when in fact most do not. It dawned on Alexander that the tightening of all the muscles in his legs and feet was part of the same habit that was causing him to tighten his neck muscles. The action of 'taking hold of the floor' with his feet had over the years become such an ingrained habit that he was completely unaware that he was doing it. He found it almost impossible to recite without all his habits being present, and whatever he did to try to change the way he recited simply increased the tension, which made things worse. Alexander's next discovery was:

A given stimulus produces the same reaction over and over again, which, if it goes unchecked, turns into habitual behaviour. This habitual reaction will eventually feel normal and natural to us.

———•———

Alexander now found himself in an impossible situation, because he needed to know what he was actually doing, but he was unable to rely on his sensory feeling kinaesthetic sense, to give him this information, because he had already found out from previous experience that it was untrustworthy.

Directions

This led Alexander to the question of how he consciously directed himself while reciting, and he realized that he never gave any thought to how he moved, but simply moved in a way that was habitual because this felt 'right' to him. Earlier I mentioned how Alexander discovered that trying to correct bad habits by deliberate action, such as pulling the head back, resulted in even more tension. So Alexander tried a different strategy: he experimented with just *thinking* of his head going forward and realized that he merely had to think of the directions in order to bring about a change. The meaning of the word *'direction'*, as Alexander used it, is consciously to give a mental order to yourself, so that you will respond to what you ask rather than working by habit alone: for example, when a person realizes that their shoulders are hunched, they think of releasing the tension and their shoulders become more relaxed. A more detailed explanation of this concept can be found later on in this book.

When Alexander had practised his directions for long enough, he decided to return to the mirrors and try out his new findings during the action of reciting. To his dismay, he found that he still failed far more often than he succeeded, yet he was sure that he was getting closer to finding an answer to his problem. He began to believe that it was his own personal shortcoming that prevented him from achieving his objectives. He looked around for all possible causes of failure. After a while he saw that he was giving his directions successfully right up to the time of reciting, but was then reverting immediately to his old habitual use of himself, pulling his head back and causing tension throughout the body. He realized that he had been so goal-oriented when it came to reciting that any attempts to 'get it right' had resulted in tension in his neck muscles: the tendency to become too focused on a goal, without considering the process required to achieve it. Alexander termed this attitude 'end-gaining', and his next challenge was to find a way to become less fixated on his goal.

Alexander decided to try giving himself a space between the stimulus to speak and the action of reciting, and he termed this course of action 'inhibition'. By giving himself this time and using his directions, he was able to notice and change the ingrained habit of pulling his head back. The principles and techniques that he conceived, which primarily consist of awareness, eradication of harmful habits and free choice, are what form the basis of what we know today as the Alexander Technique. Through diligent practice he was able not only to free himself from the harmful habits that had jeopardized his career, but also to cure himself of the recurring breathing problems that had afflicted him since birth.

Summary of Alexander's discoveries

1. Interference with our physiological mechanisms (poor posture) often occurs habitually and unconsciously.

2. The existence Primary Control, which organizes balance and co-ordination throughout the rest of oneself.

3. The way in which we use ourselves will invariably affect all of our various functions.

4. The existence of faulty sensory appreciation.

5. The body does not function as a collection of separate independent parts but as a whole unit with every part affecting every other part.

6. A given stimulus produces the same reaction over and over again, which, if it goes unchecked, turns into habitual behaviour. This habitual reaction will feel normal and natural to us.

7. Directing – to change a habit that involves muscular tension, we need to just think of what we want the muscle to do rather than actually changing it by using even more tension.

8. Inhibiting – to refuse to react to any stimulus in our automatic habitual way.

9. Eliminating 'end-gaining' – by inhibiting and directing, we can pay attention to how we perform an action and not be only thinking about the end result.

10. The mind, body and emotions are not separate entities, but act in unity with each other.

CHAPTER 3

The Development of the Technique

What you thought before has led to every choice you have made, and this adds up to you at this moment. If you want to change who you are physically, mentally, and spiritually, you will have to change what you think.

Patrick Gentempo

After his success in solving his own voice problem, Alexander abandoned his acting career and started to work with fellow actors, many of whom were suffering from similar problems. He was successful where others had failed, and the news spread like wildfire about the 'miracle healer' who had cured himself and others of a variety of ailments. Australian doctors began referring some of their patients to Alexander, and he began to gain a reputation for helping to cure many conditions previously considered incurable. He used the gentle guidance of his hands, as well as verbal instructions, to convey this new knowledge, which many people found preferable to medication or manipulation, which often had harmful side effects. He helped more and more people to change the harmful habits that were at the root of their illnesses and began to recruit other members of his family to help him with his work, in particular his brother, Albert Redden Alexander.

Some of the Australian medical profession were so convinced about the importance of Alexander's discovery for the whole of humanity that they thought Alexander should go to London to present his work to a much wider audience. A group of them, led by Dr J W Stewart McKay, a prominent Sydney surgeon, persuaded Alexander of this. So in the spring of 1904, Alexander set sail for London with letters of recommendation from several distinguished doctors and prepared himself to give lectures and speeches about his discovery of the Primary Control.

Unfortunately, however, Alexander did not receive the welcome that he or the Australian doctors had expected. In London he was seen as a threat to the medical advances that were happening at the time. Stories of the 'incurables' regaining their health and stamina at Alexander's hands only made the doctors sceptical or even hostile. Rumours went around about Alexander's 'strange hypnotic powers' and his 'peculiar personal magnetism', and many people were led to believe that he could produce temporary cures that lasted only while under Alexander's influence. The London doctors were very afraid that the honour and dignity of their distinguished profession would be threatened by a person with no qualifications. After all, Alexander had never been inside a university let alone a medical school. Unfortunately for a great many people, this irrational attitude by many in the medical profession remained for all of Alexander's lifetime.

Despite this enormous setback, Alexander went about setting up a practice, first in Victoria Street, then later at 16 Ashley Place in Central London. Gradually, as in Australia, word got out that there was a man who could help with a wide variety of often undiagnosed illnesses when no one else could. A few open-minded doctors and specialists began sending some of their patients to Alexander as a last resort when they were not responding to orthodox medical treatments. Other people approached Alexander of their own volition, because they had been told that they were incurable by the medical profession. The problems that these people presented were extremely varied and included back pain, neck problems, chronic fatigue, flat feet, voice or throat problems, nervous exhaustion, headaches, migraine, scoliosis, kyphosis, lordosis, lack of vitality, angina, rheumatism, arthritis, sleeplessness, depression, bad memory, legs of different lengths, stuttering, tennis elbow, indigestion, constipation, general unhappiness and many more.

A case history

I would like to relate the story of one of Alexander's cases to give you an idea of how he worked. An American woman known as Mrs Buchanan arrived in London in 1952 for what she called her 'final consultations', for her health had rapidly and seriously deteriorated. She had failed to recover from a recent illness and had gradually become more and more disabled. Before contracting the illness, she had always been full of energy, her appearance slender and upright, with a clear and bright complexion. Now, her head was pulled down into her shoulders, she had grown stout and round-shouldered; her skin had the look of old parchment and she could not stand without the aid of her stick. She had not walked normally for months, always dragging an ailing leg behind her. When she no longer had the energy to put on a brave face, she looked as though she was wearing a 'death mask'. She visited doctor after doctor, specialist after specialist, and faithfully followed their advice, taking all medication prescribed. The net result was, however, that she had slowly and steadily become sicker and sicker. She travelled to London as a final attempt to find a solution to her awful predicament. After more examinations and treatments over the course of three or four months in London hospitals, she overheard by chance her name being mentioned by one consultant to another. He was saying, 'Poor soul! You agree with me that there isn't a hope.'

At that point, she lost all confidence in the doctors, yet did not want to hurt their feelings as she realized that they were doing their best to help her. So she made up some excuse that she needed to return home urgently for family reasons. However, between the time that she had booked her passage and the travel date, a good friend of hers, Louise Morgan, convinced her to try to see Alexander just once before travelling home. She agreed, and within a short time she was hobbling into Alexander's teaching room for the first time, stick in hand, and was lowered gently and carefully into a chair. 'Well, here I am', she announced as cheerfully as possible. 'And only just in time', replied Alexander. 'My dear lady, you are quite the worst case of harmful use of yourself I have seen in my fifty-six years of teaching.' 'My dear sir,' she quickly retorted, 'that is not a very complimentary thing to say to a lady.' Very gently and kindly Alexander went on to explain, 'I mean that you are one mass of pressure from head to foot. Your head is pressing down on your neck and back, crushing the bones of the spine together and crushing down the muscles of your back. You have lost inches in height, I can see. You have no longer any control of the use of yourself. You are pressing yourself down all the time. Pressing down, down, down.' 'Well I never! Please tell me more', Mrs Buchanan replied, looking very interested. 'Let me show you instead', Alexander said, taking up her stick and imitating her hobble. He did it wonderfully because of his background as an actor. 'You see how I am putting down my whole weight on that stick of yours, pushing it into the ground, making terrific efforts to do so. See how it jerks my whole arm out of the shoulder and strains my back. See how it pulls my whole body out of shape. This is what you have been doing to yourself day after day. All the exercises you have been doing have only intensified the pressure. Now you know what is the matter with you. You were perhaps very ill and found it hard to walk after you got up again?' She was astounded, 'But how do you know all this?' she exclaimed, 'You haven't even examined me!' 'I diagnosed it at a glance', Alexander replied. 'You must remember I have been diagnosing people from this viewpoint for more than half a century. A wrinkle speaks volumes. The expression of the eyes can tell the whole story. Posture is a complete give-away. But don't be downhearted. You'll be throwing that horrible stick away one of these days.' Within the first lesson, to her total amazement she was able to stand up on her own two feet, something she had not been able to do for such a long time, and by the time she left for America, some 35 lessons later, she was not only back to her old self, but also taller, the colour was back in her cheeks and she was walking quite normally again. She wrote in her diary after her thirtieth lesson, 'I'm really very lucky to have found Alexander. Why doesn't everybody know

“For what it is worth I must place on record that I found in Alexander an imaginative genius and an adherence to scientific method which I have not seen out-matched by anyone. I think he transformed the human condition although as yet on a tiny scale. ”

Dr Wilfred Barlow, consultant rheumatologist and Alexander teacher

about him? This is the kind of thing we all need, I'm certain, even the healthy ones among us. It seems crazy that he should not be as famous as so many men are who don't do half what he does for the good of humanity.' The full details of her dramatic story can be found in *The Philosopher's Stone – a collection of diaries of Lessons with F. Matthias Alexander*, and *Inside Yourself* by Louise Morgan.

Influential pupils

In 1917 Alexander met the well-known American philosopher and educationist, John Dewey, while visiting America. Dewey was a prominent voice of the school of philosophy known as pragmatism and had an enormous influence on American education – in fact, he is sometimes known as 'the father of American education'.

Dewey continued taking Alexander Technique lessons for the next 35 years and was so taken by the Technique that he wrote the introductions to three of Alexander's books. In those introductions he showed his high regard for Alexander and the Technique:

> Personally, I cannot speak with too much admiration – in the original sense of wonder as well as the sense of respect – of the persistence and thoroughness with which these extremely difficult observations and experiments were carried out. In consequence, Mr Alexander created what may be truly called a physiology of the living organism. His observations and experiments have to do with the actual functioning of the body, with the organism in operation, and in operation under the ordinary conditions of living – rising, sitting, walking, standing, using arms, hands, voice, tools, instruments of all kinds.

More and more doctors were becoming convinced that Alexander's work was indeed effective, either from their own experience or from the effects that the Technique had on their patients. One of these doctors was Peter Macdonald, who in 1926 became Chairman of the Yorkshire branch of the British Medical Association. In his Inaugural Address he had this to say:

> Alexander is a teacher pure and simple. He does not profess
> to treat disease at all. If the manifestations of disease
> disappear in the process of education, well and good; if
> not, the education of itself will have been worthwhile.
> Manifestations of disease, however, do disappear. Including
> myself, I know many of his pupils, some of them, like myself
> are medical men. I have investigated some of these cases, and
> I am talking about what I know.

He went on to say that although the Technique was practically unknown to
doctors, it was of such importance that he thought that immediate investigation by the medical profession was imperative.

In 1937, a group of doctors led by Peter Macdonald wrote a letter that was
published in the *British Medical Journal*. It was signed by no fewer than 19
doctors and stated:

> As the medical men concerned we have observed the
> beneficial changes in use and functioning which have been
> brought about by the employment of Alexander's technique
> in the patients we have sent to him for help – even in the case
> of so called 'chronic disease' – whilst those of us that have
> been his pupils have personally experienced equally beneficial
> results. We are convinced that 'an unsatisfactory manner of
> use, by interfering with general functioning, constitutes a pre-
> disposing cause of disorder and disease,' and that diagnosis
> of a patient's troubles must remain incomplete unless the
> medical man when making his diagnosis takes into consider-
> ation the influence of use upon functioning.
>
> Unfortunately, those responsible for the selection of
> subjects to be studied by medical students have not yet inves-
> tigated the new field of knowledge and experience which
> has been opened up through Alexander's work, otherwise
> we believe that ere now the training necessary for acquiring
> this knowledge would have been included in the medical
> curriculum. To this end we beg to urge that as soon as

possible steps should be taken for an investigation of Alexander's work and Technique...

Unfortunately, due to the outbreak of the Second World War, all follow-up to this letter was abandoned.

Alexander also helped the famous author Aldous Huxley, when his poor physical state threatened to end his writing career. Huxley came to see Alexander after he had been suffering from chronic fatigue, insomnia and a weak stomach. He was virtually bedridden and had been reduced to writing lying down with his typewriter resting on his chest. Learning and applying the principles of the Alexander Technique enabled him to resume his normal activities and live a good healthy life for another quarter-century. He was so impressed with the changes in his health that Alexander helped him achieve that he became a strong supporter of the work and referred to the principles of the Technique many times in his later writings; he even based a character ('Miller') in his 1936 novel *Eyeless in Gaza* on Alexander. Huxley firmly believed that the Alexander Technique was a 'totally new type of education, affecting the entire range of human activity, from a physiological through the intellectual, moral, and practical to the spiritual' and was not afraid to publicize the fact.

Many other prominent members of society at the time sought Alexander's help, including Sir Charles Sherrington, Chancellor of the Exchequer Sir Stafford Cripps, Lord Lytton and the Archbishop of Canterbury, William Temple. Alexander continued to help many thousands of people until shortly before his death in October 1955.

It is hard to believe that even today the validity of Alexander's work is largely unacknowledged, despite public recognition by many internationally recognized scientists and doctors (*see* the science and medicine quotations throughout the book). The fact is that although Alexander himself had no medical training and no access to medical diagnostic tests and equipment, and despite the fact that he never prescribed medication, exercises or treatment of any kind, nevertheless, time and time again he succeeded in helping people back to health where science and medicine had failed.

CHAPTER 4

How the Alexander Technique Works

Alexander established not only the beginnings of a far reaching science of the apparently involuntary movements we call reflexes, but a technique of correction and self-control which forms a substantial addition to our very slender resources in personal education.

George Bernard Shaw

The Alexander Technique is simple to understand, yet it does take time to learn. Alexander said that even a child of three could learn it. In fact, children learn more quickly than most adults, because they have far fewer detrimental habits to lose. As described in chapter 2, Alexander's problem with his voice was largely one of posture. He was holding himself in a rigid way, gripping the floor with his feet and pulling his head back with a great deal of force. Everything he tried *to do* to solve his problem did not work; it was only when he could see what he was doing wrong and was able to *stop doing it* that he made any progress. Alexander was a very practical man and he had little time for theories that were not tested in a practical way, and because of this his technique is very down-to-earth and can be easily comprehended by anyone willing to put in the time to learn it. The only requirement is that you approach it with an open mind, patience and a willingness to learn about your own unconscious habits.

Habitual behaviour

When initially attempting to learn the Alexander Technique, many people get the wrong idea. This is because people often assume that there is a 'correct' posture; a correct way of walking, standing and sitting. Yet this is as far away from the Technique as you can get. Alexander once said:

> Boiled down, it all comes to inhibiting a particular reaction
> to a given stimulus. But no one will see it that way. They
> will see it as getting in and out of a chair the right way. It is
> nothing of the kind. It is that a pupil decides what he will or
> will not consent to do.

It is important to understand that the Alexander Technique involves not so much learning as *unlearning*. It is a practical way of releasing the unnecessary and harmful muscular tension that you may have accumulated unconsciously over many years.

Many of the postural habits that we acquire in life are harmful to our health because they involve exerting excessive and unnecessary muscle tension in every action we do. Unfortunately, most of us are totally unaware of this tension, even though others can often see it clearly. Just watch a typical adult getting off the sofa and notice the great effort often involved in this very simple task. By gradually becoming aware and reducing the level of tension in your body, we will be able to achieve a better posture and a much more graceful way of moving. This relieves or prevents many common aches and pains, and allows unrestricted functioning of the respiratory, circulatory and digestive systems. Since the way we feel physically affects our mental and emotional outlook on life, releasing muscular tension also helps us to become calmer and generally happier in our day-to-day lives.

Many people think of the Alexander Technique as just another relaxation technique, but it is nothing of the kind. Although you will learn how to reduce the tension in some of the muscles that have become tense, other muscles may in fact have to *increase* in tone. It is a method that brings the entire muscular and reflex system back into balance. You will also learn new and easier ways of moving while performing everyday tasks, which will result in far less strain on you. You will discover ways of sitting, standing and walking that put less strain on the bones, joints and muscles, allowing your body to work more effectively and efficiently. In fact, many people who

5: Even simple activities such as ironing can cause stress on the whole body if the head is not balanced easily on top of the spine.

6: In contrast to the woman in photo 5, this person's head is more balanced and therefore there is less strain on the rest of the body.

practise the Technique experience a general feeling of lightness throughout their bodies and have even described the sensation as like 'walking on air'. One of my pupils described the feeling after an Alexander lesson as the 'champagne feeling', because she felt light and bubbly. Since our physical state directly affects our mental and emotional wellbeing, people often say that they feel much calmer and happier after even just a few Alexander lessons, often resulting in less domestic tension and a greater ability to cope with life in general.

The Alexander Technique also involves examining and improving posture, breathing, balance and coordination, which are inseparable from one another. As children, our posture, while we are still or in movement, is a joy to watch, but as we start to tense our muscles in reaction to many of life's worries and concerns, our posture deteriorates into what can eventually border on deformity. Anyone can see that most children have a better posture and move more gracefully than adults. Yet this is normally not the case with people outside the developed countries – many of the indigenous races who still live on the land, such as the Berber people from North Africa, the Native Americans from North America or the Aborigines in Australia, retain their natural posture throughout their lives.

Children do not 'do' anything to have good posture. It is all done for them by the brain's automatic mechanisms and responses. They have a series of reflexes throughout the body that provide support and natural coordination of their movements without any conscious effort on their part. So do we adults – the only difference being that as adults we interfere with these natural reflexes, because many of us hold far more tension than is good for us. In fact, without realizing it, many of us make life much harder for ourselves than it really needs to be and this adversely affects posture. Our shoulders become permanently hunched, our necks become stiffer and stiffer, and we sit either slumped or holding ourselves in a very rigid fashion. As our minds become more and more concerned with the future and the past, and our awareness of the present moment diminishes, we start to lose awareness of how we stand, sit and move.

It is often hard for us to detect this increase in tension because it builds up gradually over the years. We become accustomed to the ways in which we sit and stand, and while these ways may feel comfortable to us, they are often putting strain upon our body without our realizing it. No matter how

7: One of the reasons that many people suffer with back pain after vacuuming is that they bend their back instead of their knees. As a consequence, the lower back muscles are under considerable strain because they are supporting the entire weight of the upper body while it is bent forward.

8: In comparison to the woman in photo 7, this person is doing the same task of vacuuming , but is much more upright, and as a result her muscles are not under the same stress.

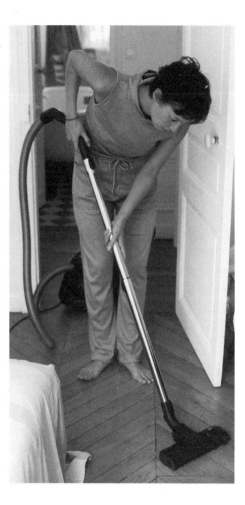

9: When bending down, young children naturally bend their hip, knee and ankle joints and keep there back align.

10: In contrast to the child in photo 9, adults in developed countries rarely bend their hip, knee and ankle joints, but bend their backs instead. This can result in a multitude of musculo-skeletal problems.

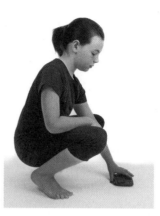

uncoordinated these positions become, they will feel right to us. In the end, poor posture, or as Alexander called it, 'misuse', will feel comfortable and 'right' and good posture (similar to the original natural posture we had as a young child) will initially feel strange and wrong. This is the effect of what Alexander termed 'faulty sensory appreciation'.

It may not be until years later that we start to suffer from aches and pains or restriction of movement, so, crucially, we often do not make the connection that our poor posture or misuse of ourselves is responsible for the pain. Contemporary methods of combating such problems typically involve powerful painkilling or anti-inflammatory drugs, or muscle relaxants, but these can block out the body's warning system, whose function it is to tell us that something is wrong. Often, doctors can offer little advice because their training centres on treating symptoms rather than uncovering, and rectifying, the actual causes of such problems.

The Alexander Technique, however, does the opposite. It can show you the underlying causes, so that you are then able to eliminate the tension responsible for many of the ailments that are so often mistakenly put down to the ageing process. To illustrate this, consider the true story of a 55-year-old lady who came to me with a problem with her left leg. Her leg gave her a great deal of pain whenever she stood or walked on it. She had approached her doctor who sent her for tests and an X-ray. When the results came through, the doctor told the lady that she had arthritis, that this was caused by normal 'wear and tear', and that, as she was getting on in years, she needed to accept this problem. The lady refused to believe that the reason was simply wear and tear alone because, as she pointed out to her doctor, her right leg was perfectly all right and as far as she was aware both of her legs were exactly the same age! When she started having Alexander lessons, we quickly discovered that she had a habit of always standing on her left leg, and this was obviously putting excessive strain on it. Over the course of her lessons she became aware of what she was doing and made a conscious choice to change the way she used herself, and as a result she started to stand evenly on both feet. When she did this, the pain was immediately reduced, and within a few weeks she was walking and standing without any pain whatsoever.

Back pain

One of the most common examples of how posture can affect our health is back pain. According to the UK-based charity BackCare, on average a third of people living in industrialized countries suffer from back pain at any given time, and a staggering 80 per cent of the population of these countries will have disabling back pain at some point in their lives. The Health and Safety Executive in the UK agrees that back pain will affect as many as four-fifths of people during their lifetime and results in 4.5 million working days lost each year. In the US, the National Center for Health Statistics reports very similar percentages. They say that over 76 million people in the US are suffering with backache at any given moment.

Statistics reveal that back pain is on the increase in most industrialized countries, yet there are no clear solutions to the problem in the established medical sciences. Although large sums of money are being spent on treatment of the pain, often with unpleasant side effects, there is little research into why back pain is so prevalent in industrialized countries, yet comparatively rare in developing countries. Doctors, back specialists and orthopaedic surgeons will often openly admit that the cause of back pain is frequently a mystery, and the same can be said for other ailments, such as arthritis, asthma or headaches. My father, who was a family doctor, used to say that if you want a day off work, you should just say you have back problems, because nobody can prove you have, and nobody can prove you haven't, and even if you have, nobody can do anything about it. This was certainly true of my own back problem, and it was the reason I first became involved with the Alexander Technique.

My story

I came to the Technique through back pain. This was primarily caused by poor posture due to my sedentary profession as a driving instructor. My posture was so hunched that a person once said that I looked like someone who had been living in a *very* small cottage with *very* low ceilings for a *very* long time! I often spent over 50 hours a week sitting in a car, and after several years at the job I developed lower back pain. At first it was an occasional aching back that was relieved by massage or some gentle exercise, but before long I was suffering with such a very painful condition that I could hardly walk. I did not know it at the time, but my search to try and get relief for my painful and debilitating condition would take me on an incredible journey of self-discovery.

The first port of call was my father, who was a medical doctor, and although he was obviously very concerned about my condition, he could offer me little help apart from painkillers and the usual (in those days) medical advice of rest. This brought only temporary relief, and as time went by even the powerful painkilling drugs I was taking became less and less effective. It was not long before I needed to get back to work due to financial pressures, but sitting in the car only made the problem worse.

Medical treatment

I then attended several physiotherapists over a number of years, and although some of the treatments helped for a day or two, my condition got steadily worse and worse. Before long I was also suffering with sciatic pains that were shooting down my left leg, and I got to a stage where I could not sit, stand or walk without pain shooting through my whole body.

Eventually, after a long wait, I saw a series of back specialists who took X-rays and performed various other tests. Although a prolapsed disc was diagnosed as the cause of my problem, no one could tell me what had caused the disc to move out of position in the first place, or how I could get it back in place. I was only told that I would have to get used to the fact that I would never be able to live a normal life again and that I should avoid bending, lifting and carrying anything at all costs. The surgeon advised me to undergo surgery to remove the three lowest intervertebral discs, because this, I was promised, would reduce the level of pain. I initially agreed to this, but then my father persuaded me to cancel the operation because he was treating people who had undergone similar operations, many of whom were in even more pain than before, and very few were actually any better. So as a last desperate attempt to find some relief from the pain I underwent an intensive course of physiotherapy treatment as an inpatient at a large residential phys-iotherapy hospital near London, UK. One of the treatments at the hospital involved improving posture, and I was told 'hold yourself straight' and 'pull your shoulders back', but this only aggravated my pain instantly; in fact, it aggravated the problem of all the other patients in the session too.

Although the physiotherapists were obviously doing their best to help, the treatment and exercises they gave were not helping me at all; in fact, when I was discharged from the hospital my back pain was worse than ever.

Alternative treatments

At this stage I started to investigate various forms of alternative medicine. These included the more established therapies, such as chiropractic, osteopathy, homeopathy and acupuncture, and then I tried less orthodox treatments, such as reflexology, metamorphic technique, aromatherapy, Reiki and spiritual healing. In fact, I was so desperate I would have tried practically anything, and while some of these treatments helped to some extent, I could still get only short-term relief, as the severe pain always returned within days of any treatment. I finally gave up after many years of searching and resigned myself to a life of pain. Up to this point no one, including myself, had considered why the discs had become prolapsed in the first place.

By chance one day I met an Alexander teacher by the name of Danny Reilly, who explained that the Alexander Technique could be very effective in helping back sufferers like myself who had tried many other remedies without success. Although I had no idea what it was, and was understandably very sceptical after all the other treatments I had received, I decided to have a couple of sessions to see what it was all about. At this point I was quite desperate as the pain was present day and night and so I felt that I had nothing to lose. I had no idea what 'learning the Alexander Technique' meant. As I had come across the Technique in the context of music and acting, being neither a musician nor an actor, I was not sure how it was going to help me.

During my first lesson, within minutes Danny asked me whether I always sat the way I was sitting. I replied that I really did not understand what he was talking about, so he put a mirror in front of me and I could see that I was twisting to the right while leaning at least 20 degrees to the left. Yet despite the fact that I was obviously sitting in a very crooked way, I felt perfectly straight. This was quite a revelation to me. I was amazed that I (or anyone else) had never noticed it before. Danny set about making a few gentle adjustments to the way I was sitting and two things happened: in my new position I felt completely twisted to the left and leaning way off to the right, yet at the same time my back pain started to ease. He showed me how I was now sitting in the mirror and to my amazement I saw with my own eyes that I was sitting perfectly straight.

After a few lessons, the changes felt less strange and my back pain slowly but surely started to abate. It was at this point that I realized that when I had been teaching people to drive, I had developed the habit of leaning to the left while twisting my pelvis to the right; this was so that I could see both the road ahead and check to make sure that the learner driver was looking in the mirrors at the same time. Over the years this had become my habit whenever I sat, and it was this very habit that had given me all my problems. As the tensions released more and more during a series of lessons, I also noticed that it was not only my back that was improving: I also started to sleep better, my self-esteem and confidence grew and, to my surprise, I was gradually becoming happier as well. Within three months I was leading a normal life again and was lifting and bending without any problem at all.

Many people carry on, as I did, for years with unnecessary pain, not realizing that anything can be done about it. We do, however, need to face up to the fact that we have to take responsibility for our ailments and not expect others to have all the answers. The Technique opens up a journey of personal discovery. Pain is simply the body's warning system, trying to tell us that something is wrong. If heeded, it will urge us to consider our posture and the way we move our bodies while performing even the simplest of tasks. If you were driving a car and the oil light came on, you would not take out the bulb and carry on driving; this, of course, would be foolish. You would stop the car and endeavour to find what was wrong, and if you did not you could expect more serious problems later. Yet we are not encouraged to apply the same logic to the body. Many ways of treating back problems today are, in effect, attempts to eliminate pain without investigating what is causing it in the first place.

Since the physical postures we tend to adopt are actually a reflection of our inner state, many people find that when learning the Alexander Technique, they also become aware of, and can begin to change, the mental and emotional habits that have been present for most of their lives. When learning the technique you will begin to recognize behaviour patterns that are no longer serving you and this will help you to gain a new self-awareness and freedom of choice. This naturally leads to a greater inner harmony that will be reflected in your posture. So when applying the Alexander

Technique as a daily practice, you will be able to make conscious choices not only in the physical sense but also on many levels, allowing you to have more freedom in every aspect of your life.

Alexander lessons

Because it is often extremely difficult to see your own habits and areas of tension, finding a teacher is very important to help you through the difficulties that will often arise during the learning process. Although, of course, Alexander himself did solve his own problems without any help from others, he did take a great deal of time and a lot of determination to do so, and he was a pioneer in the field. Most of us today would not choose to spend all that time identifying our harmful habits without the help and guidance of a trained Alexander Technique teacher.

In this book you will learn about the principles and the philosophy behind the Alexander Technique, but it is not a substitute for actual lessons from a qualified teacher: after all, you would not expect to drive a car after only reading a teach-yourself-to-drive book. Having studied the principles of the Technique explained in this book, however, you will be able to understand more easily and quickly what your teacher is trying to convey, saving you both time and money. A good understanding of the principles will also help you to take responsibility for your learning process.

Learning the Alexander Technique consists of four stages:

1. Becoming aware of all postural habits that cause or exacerbate a lack of coordination and a general misuse of yourself.

2. Releasing the unwanted tension accumulated over many years of standing, moving or sitting in an uncoordinated manner.

3. Learning new ways of moving, standing or sitting that are easier and more efficient and that put less stress on the body, thus reducing excessive wear and tear on the bones and joints as well as allowing all the internal organs space to function naturally.

4. Learning new ways of reacting physically, emotionally and mentally to various situations.

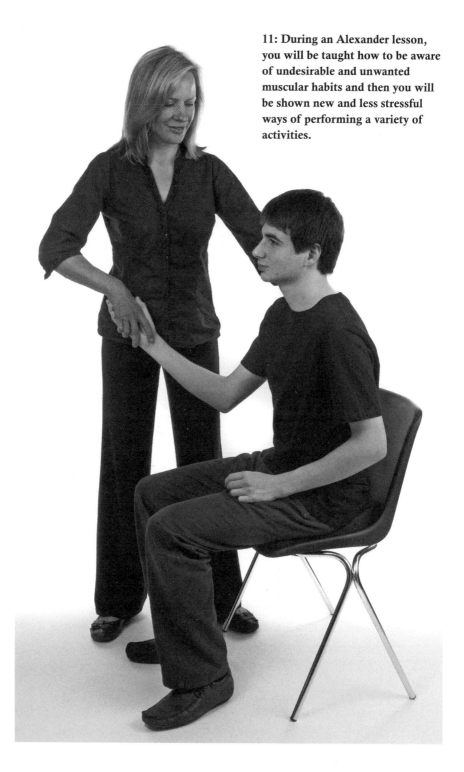

11: During an Alexander lesson, you will be taught how to be aware of undesirable and unwanted muscular habits and then you will be shown new and less stressful ways of performing a variety of activities.

12: The freedom of the neck is of primary importance, for without it the head cannot balance freely on top of the spine, which is essential for good posture One of the first things an Alexander teacher usually shows you is how to release the tension in the neck.

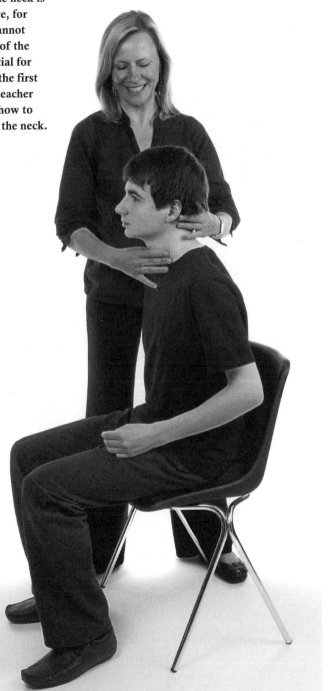

You are never too old to learn the Technique! As previously outlined, I have taught people well into their eighties who have made remarkable progress. However, of course the younger you are, the fewer habits you will have accumulated and therefore it is likely that you will be able to change the harmful habits more quickly.

An Alexander Technique lesson typically lasts between 30 and 60 minutes. During this time your teacher will gently move you to see if he or she can detect places where you may be holding muscular tension. The process is very gentle and painless. When tension is discovered, your teacher will ask you to notice and, if you can, to let go of it, and you may be amazed at the difference in how you feel after only a few lessons.

Awareness

The key to learning the Technique is awareness. It may seem a little odd at first to make an effort to become aware of how we perform various tasks, because many of our movements have become automatic and we tend to perform them over and over again in the same way without conscious thought. Gradually, though, we learn to think briefly before performing any given action to see if it can be carried out with much less tension.

Once this awareness is achieved, very often we will realize how we have been causing our muscles to over-tense needlessly every time we move. By analysing even simple movements, such as walking or getting up from a chair, we can find new ways of moving that releases muscular tension rather than creating it. People who have undergone a course of lessons often experience less tiredness and have more energy to do the things they enjoy. Their quality of life is greatly enhanced, and feelings of calm, happiness and greater wellbeing begin to replace feelings of exhaustion or anxiety.

Re-education

When you begin to apply the principles of the Technique, you will not be learning anything new, but simply unlearning the bad habits you have acquired during the course of your life. Alexander often said that if you stopped doing the wrong thing (i.e. the habit), the right thing would happen by itself, and this principle is at the very heart of the Technique. It is, however, sometimes harder to relearn it than it is to learn something in the first place, because our usual way of performing actions always feels so right to us. As we start to allow tension to release, we find that we are naturally using ourselves in a much more balanced and coordinated way without any effort.

It is important to realize that the whole process of re-evaluating the way in which we stand, sit and move does take time, as we are dealing with habits that have probably been present since childhood. These days we have come to expect immediate results, and yet nature is not like that: it will take time for posture to change. We even have habits in the way we think, and in the process of learning the Alexander Technique we begin to be aware of how our minds sometimes get in the way of this change. As part of the process, we begin to catch the harmful habits of both body and mind, so change can be profound and multifaceted.

Changing patterns of behaviour

We have all developed physical, mental and emotional patterns of behaviour that we take for granted, and it is often easier for others to see these when we ourselves cannot. We react to a given situation over and over again in a set way, irrespective of whether it is appropriate. We make certain assumptions, and these influence our choices and reactions, yet in many cases we are unaware that we are doing this. As a result, we repeat them time after time. Many of these ways of responding were learnt in childhood, some even before our earliest memory, so they obviously feel totally normal to us. Bringing these habits to consciousness with the help of the Technique can help us become freer, happier and more conscious human beings.

  ❝ I find the Alexander Technique very helpful in my work. Things happen without you trying. They get to be light and relaxed. You must get an Alexander teacher to show it to you. ❞

John Cleese, comedian and actor

51

Summary of the chapter:

The Alexander Technique is:

- A way of becoming aware and letting go of tension throughout your body.

- A re-education, so that you learn how to use your body in a more appropriate way, and thus avoid putting stress on the bones, joints and internal organs.

- A process in which you will get to know yourself better.

- A way of making real choices in your life, rather than reacting habitually and unconsciously to any given situation.

- A way of understanding how you are naturally designed to work, and how to stop interfering with your body's natural functions.

- A technique that you will immediately be able to use in daily life to bring about greater harmony and contentment.

CHAPTER 5

Understanding Posture

A correct position or posture indicates a fixed position, and a person held to a fixed position cannot grow, as we understand growth. The correct position today cannot be the correct position a week later for any person who is advancing in the work of re-education and coordination.

F Matthias Alexander

Ida Rolf, the originator of 'Rolfing', once said 'The minute you use force to maintain a certain posture, you betray that all is not well with your world. You show the world that your structure and your posture are at war.' As a result of this force and tension, there are a great many people today that are literally 'sick and tired' because of the detrimental effects of poor posture. It could be a back or neck problem, shallow breathing or just a feeling of constant tiredness. Many do not know where to start in order to improve posture and feel frustrated that any attempt to improve things proves ineffective or short-lived. If you are one of those people who would like a posture that is beautifully balanced with graceful coordination, but have been unsuccessful in your efforts in trying to obtain it, please read on, because this chapter will help to dispel many of the misconceptions there are around posture and how to improve it.

As previously discussed, poor posture not only leaves you exhausted at the end of the day, but also can cause or exacerbate a wide range of muscular problems, poor breathing habits and stiff joints. It can also be associated with low self-esteem or depression. In fact, undesirable posture can hold you back in nearly every aspect of your life. In contrast, good posture can say a lot about a person. People who have a naturally upright alignment appear taller, are more attractive and graceful and exude subtle confidence.

When people find out that I teach the Alexander Technique, I find that many of them immediately sit bolt upright, arch their backs and pull their shoulders back, thinking that they have now improved their posture. This is because so many people have been taught 'to sit up straight' in their childhood, but that is not what the Alexander Technique is about at all; in fact, it is quite the opposite. Posture is far more complex than just standing or sitting up straight; it can be described as the way in which we support and balance our bodies against the ever-present force of gravity while we go about our daily activities. The human body is truly an amazing anti-gravity mechanism, yet most of us unconsciously interfere with its natural workings to such an extent that we practically paralyse the muscle we are trying to use. I think this interference is the main reason why millions of people in industrialized countries suffer from muscular-related ailments such as back pain, neck problems and stiff joints.

Posture training

As we have seen, the most common way that we try to improve our posture is by pulling in our lower backs when sitting or standing 'up straight', or drastically over-tensing the shoulder and upper back muscles as we try to 'pull our shoulders back'. It is quite apparent to others that we are working the muscsles too hard and doing far too much and will not be able to maintain this posture for long, but for us it is practically the only way we were taught to improve posture as children.

Although the instruction to 'sit/stand up straight' was the most common postural training instruction we were given, it does not improve anything – in fact, it really only makes things worse. I find that when people first come to me to try and change their postural habits, many of them often find it difficult *not* to sit up straight with an over-arched lumbar curve. This is not because it is hard, as in reality it is far easier, but because it is the exact

13: When trying to 'improve our posture' by standing up straight, we are often only making the problem worse, because by doing so we often add even more tension to a muscle system that is already under strain.

14: In stark contrast, a child is naturally straight and is not 'doing' anything to be straight. All other systems throughout the body are allowed to work without hindrance, thus maintaining good health.

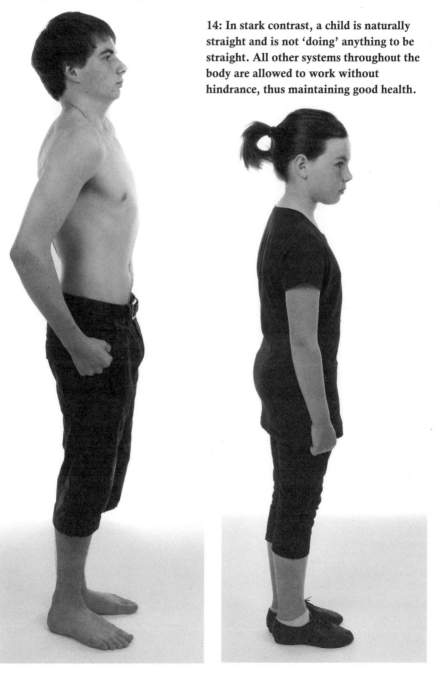

opposite of what they have been taught all their lives. The habit of over-arching the back has become so ingrained that, for many people, it actually feels wrong not to do it. This detrimental posture training is often given to children at a time when they are easily influenced and do not question the instructions given to them. I think that this is the main reason that most people still think improving posture means forcing or tensing the body into different shapes. Very few people have been given the tools they need to effectively improve their posture, which is what I hope to convey throughout this book. It is, in fact, a fresh approach to improving posture naturally – a way that does not involve physical effort and a method that everyone can learn.

Defining posture

Before we start trying to improve our posture, it is important to take a moment in order to get clear on what exactly it is we are trying to improve. This is perhaps more complex than it first seems, because many people can easily describe 'good posture' or 'bad posture', but find it much more difficult to accurately explain the word *posture* on its own or understand how good posture can be achieved effectively. When asked to define the word 'posture', most people describe it in one of the following ways:

- The position of my body during various activities

- The way in which I hold my body

- The shape that I am in at any given time

- The way I hold myself

- The way I carry myself

- My body's position or stance

- The position of my limbs and body as a whole

- The way that I am

- The way that I hold my body when standing, sitting or moving

- The way I place my body and limbs

❛❛ I was dubious about the effects of the Alexander
Technique when I first went in to experience it, but I
found out almost immediately that the benefits were
total – both physically and mentally – and, happily,
have also been long-lasting. ❜❜

Joanne Woodward, actress

Just think for a moment – which one of these descriptions do you identify
with? When someone thinks of improving their posture, they generally
think of getting a better shape or position, and when they describe their own
posture usually the words *'hold'*, *'position'* and *'shape'* come to mind. However,
when we think of someone who already has good posture, many people think
of a young child playing or an African woman walking so gracefully carrying
a heavy water jar on top of her head. In both cases there is free and graceful
movement that has little to do with *holding, shape* or *position*.

It is also interesting to note that when people are describing their own
posture, the phrase that is most often repeated is *'the way* I hold myself' or
'the way I sit and stand'. This is because in developed countries most adults
have lost the variety of natural movement that they had as children: a posture
that is upright yet free, one that involves lots of different shapes and
movements. 'The way' simply describes the stereotyped habits that we have
adopted. Just watch young children in any school playground – they are
skipping, then hopping, walking on their heels, then walking on tip-toe.
Their movements are constantly changing and they do not have a 'set' way of
sitting, standing or moving. In sharp contrast, most adults hold themselves in
unnatural stances and have very definite stereotyped postural patterns of
movement. These habitual patterns of movement are easily identifiable to
others, but not to themselves. So it can be difficult to recognize your own
small child at a distance when playing on a beach by the way he or she
moves, because the way they are moving is constantly varying; instead, you
have to identify them by the colour of the clothes they are wearing. Yet, you can
easily recognize your adult friends by *the way* they walk, even before you

can recognize their faces or clothing. These postural habits that we have unconsciously adopted can affect mobility and can even lead to physical disability and pain; this is entirely due to the excessive muscular tension that any fixed posture produces.

Alexander did not like the word 'posture' and used it as little as possible, because he found it too restrictive and did not consider the mind and emotions that also need to be taken into account. He also realized that many of us associated posture with a static condition – something that they were taught at school, rather than a dynamic, vibrant and natural way of being that we were born with. He could even see with his own pupils that they were trying to 'get something' rather than let go of their habits that affected the way that they used themselves as a whole, and once said: 'You are not here to do exercises or to learn something right, but to get able to meet a stimulus that always puts you wrong and learn to deal with it.' Many of us do not even recognize that we have particular habits that are affecting our posture let alone know how to refrain from doing them.

Redefining posture

So it is important to understand that posture is not merely a position or shape: it is our response to gravity at any given moment. There is no single correct way to stand or sit, even though I am sure most people would agree that there are potentially harmful ways of doing so. Natural posture is the product of a set of innate reflexes, called the 'postural reflexes', which maintain balance and good coordination, without any conscious involvement on your part. If you begin to lose your balance, your postural reflexes go into operation immediately and put you upright again. These reflexes are totally automatic and are activated by various reflex 'triggers' throughout your body, yet without knowing, we often interfere in their operation by holding much more muscular tension than we need. This tension is the direct result of the unconscious postural habits and inappropriate stereotyped ways of moving that we have been talking about.

A more accurate definition of the word *posture* is:

The relationship of one or more parts of the body to the rest.

When that relationship is free, good posture happens naturally, but when that relationship is restricted because of tension, poor posture is inevitable, irrespective of the position or shape we adopt. In summary, if we have freedom within the body, the right posture will be there without us having to do anything. To achieve this we need to start to become aware of, and let go of, the unnecessary and unconscious tension that we carry.

Postural reflexes and muscles

When looking at how the muscular system works, it is important to realize that there are two very different types of muscle, which are responsible for doing two very different jobs. There are the muscles that organize *posture* and those that organize *movement*. While it is true that any muscles can at times do both tasks, some muscles are more suited to the task of performing movement while others the task of maintaining posture.

The first type of muscle, whose primary task is to keep us upright against the ever-present force of gravity, is often referred to as the *postural muscle*. We rarely have to think about maintaining our balance as we go about our daily activities – it is all done for us by an amazing system of complex postural reflexes without any conscious effort on our part. We can stand for a long time without these muscles tiring because they are 'fatigue resistant' and are automatically triggered by powerful reflexes throughout the body, producing the appropriate muscle tone. As soon as the stimulus for these reflexes is reduced, these muscles automatically relax. We are often not aware of these processes because they often take place below the level of our consciousness.

By contrast, the *phasic muscles*, which are more suited to perform activities, work very differently: if you want to raise an arm, you must first make a conscious decision to move the arm and then determine how much you want to lift it. The muscles you use in this way react quickly, but also tire quickly. You can try this for yourself by holding your arm out to your side horizontally; within a few minutes you will be able to feel the muscles in your arm begin to tire. This becomes clearer when you look at the chart overleaf, which compares the different types of muscle and their function.

The crucial point here is that trying to improve posture by deliberately sitting up straight and pulling our shoulders back will never ever work, no matter how hard we try, because we will be using our phasic muscles rather

POSTURAL MUSCLES	PHASIC MUSCLES
These muscles are designed to keep us upright	These muscles are primarily designed to perform actions.
The primary function of these muscles is to support and keep us balanced against the force of gravity.	We use these muscles primarily to perform movements.
They have a predominance of muscle fibres that are *reddish* in colour.	They have a predominance of muscle fibres that are *whitish* in colour.
These red fibres contract relatively slowly and are referred to as 'slow twitch'.	These white fibres contract quickly and are referred to as 'fast twitch'.
These muscles are fatigue resistant and therefore take a very long time to tire.	These muscles are not fatigue resistant and therefore tire quickly.
These muscles are activated by our postural reflexes and therefore do not need the conscious mind to activate them.	These muscles are activated by the conscious mind.

than our postural muscles to do so. They are simply not the right muscles for the job and as a result will tire very quickly, and so we will not be able to maintain even what we think is a 'good position' for very long. So, even with the best of intentions, if we use the 'phasic muscles' to improve our posture (which is exactly what most of us do when we try to 'improve posture'), we will fail time and time again, and we will soon find ourselves with exactly the same postural problems that we had when we started. Even if someone had lots of willpower and was prepared to put up with the discomfort, over time these muscles would become fatigued and gradually become more and more immobile, eventually causing one of the many musculoskeletal problems that we see today.

Instead, the key to good posture is to learn to reduce the amount of tension in the overworked phasic muscles so that the postural muscles will automatically start to work as they were designed to do. This is what Alexander meant when he said that if you stop the wrong thing, the right thing will happen by itself. How to let go of inappropriate muscle tension will be explained in later chapters.

There is also another point to consider: muscles are able to perform only two actions: they can contract (become shorter) or stop contracting (become longer). Muscles generally work in pairs: one muscle will contract and the other will lengthen to produce movement. If your shoulders are rounded, then it is the muscles in the front of the body (for example, the pectoralis major) that are over-contracted; this has the effect that the shoulders are pulled forward. Because muscles can only contract or stop contracting, it is obvious that the problem lies with the front muscles, yet instead of trying to find a way of releasing the front muscles, many people try to rectify the situation by deliberately pulling the shoulders back, which is merely contracting a completely different set of muscles in the upper back (for example, the latissimus dorsi). So, in effect, the front and back muscles are working against each other like a 'tug of war', and this can dramatically affect the free movement of the shoulder. This example illustrates how all too often our attempts to 'improve our posture' actually result in more muscular tension, which only makes matters worse, rather than better. Again, Alexander's statement 'When you stop doing the wrong thing, the right thing does itself' is particularly apt when it comes to improving posture in the above situation. If we can learn to release the over-tightened front muscles, the shoulder will return to its natural state. Dr Miriam Wohl, an Alexander Teacher and medical doctor, summed up the issue nicely: 'When we use constructive conscious control, by applying the Alexander principles, we can employ our thinking abilities to elicit our postural reflexes and to refrain from using the phasic muscles to support us, and making our posture more natural.'

Mind, body and emotional unity

There is another way of describing posture:

It is the outward expression of how you feel inside.

A good example of this is watching the posture of a player who has just won a sports match, compared with the player who has just lost. The one who has just won naturally has an open and upright look, while the one who has lost

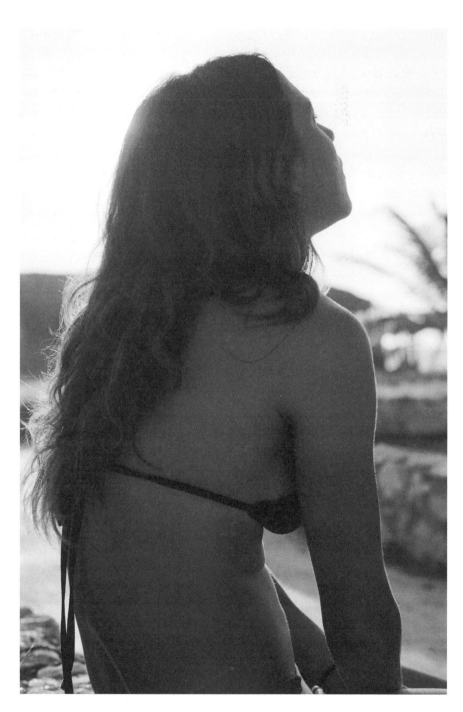

15: Just as the body, mind and emotions are one, so the way we sit, stand or move directly affects the way we think and feel.

often has rounded shoulders and a 'pulled down' look about them. So, it is important to realize that when we begin to change the way we think we will be also bringing about physical and emotional changes too.

Another example can be seen when observing a person who suffers from depression. Although depression is seen by many as a mental or emotional illness, it is clearly portrayed by the outward shape of the person. They are actually physically 'pulled down' or 'depressed' by muscular tension. It is interesting that the word 'depress', which we use to describe an emotional or mental state, can also be applied to a physical thing such as a cardboard box.

Since the mind and body are inseparable, adopting a rigid position or shape also affects the way we think or feel, because a tense body reflects rigid thinking, pain or the suppression of emotions. Poor posture can also be caused by the way we think. Our thoughts are powerful enough to produce a physical or emotional reaction, and often we feel that we can do little about it. In order to start to improve our posture, it is essential that we treat the body, mind and emotions as a whole and not look upon them as separate entities. Thousands of years ago, the famous Greek physician, Hippocrates, stated that the treatment of physical symptoms without consideration of the patient's mental and emotional state would be completely ineffective. The same applies to our posture. Yet today, when trying to improve posture, it is often only our physical symptoms that are given consideration; we do not usually take into account our mental or emotional state. This is partly due to the views of the French philosopher René Descartes, who believed that the mind and body were made of different substances and were therefore governed by different laws. His theory of mind–body division has dominated science for nearly 400 years, and it is only in the last few years that neuroscientists are realizing that the mind and body are truly indivisible, and therefore improving posture must involve improving the way we use our whole self and not just the physical body.

So, the first thing we need to do to achieve a healthier, more natural posture is to realize that we never have to 'sit up straight' again! Instead, we need to find out what caused our posture to *deteriorate* in the first place and eliminate this from our lives. We will start in the next chapter to examine one of the biggest reasons why we obtain poor posture in the first place: the classroom.

CHAPTER 6

Posture and Education

The Kinaesthetic Systems concerned with correct and
healthy bodily movements and postures have become
demoralized by the habits engendered in the
schoolroom through the restraint enforced at a time
when natural activity should have been encouraged and
scientifically directed, and in the crouching positions
necessitated by useless and irrational deskwork.

F Matthias Alexander

While listening to an educational programme on the radio recently, I heard
the Principal of a school express his concern about the changes he saw in
children during their school years. He reported that he saw children aged four
or five arriving each morning with bright eyes, smiling faces, beautiful posture
and ease of movement; they were nearly always talkative, eager to please,
willing to learn, with a playful nature, and generally enthusiastic about life.
By the time these same children left the school in their late teens, however, he
noticed that they hardly looked anyone in the eye, their posture was very
stooped, they had developed rounded shoulders and hunched backs, they were
often lazy and uninterested in the environment around them and they generally
looked unhappy. 'What', he was asking, 'in the name of education are we
doing to our children to make them change so dramatically?'

That is a very important question to ask, but unfortunately for the children
not many people ask it. In the early 1950s an investigation was carried out in
London on 892 girls and 960 boys aged between 2 and 17 years of age. The

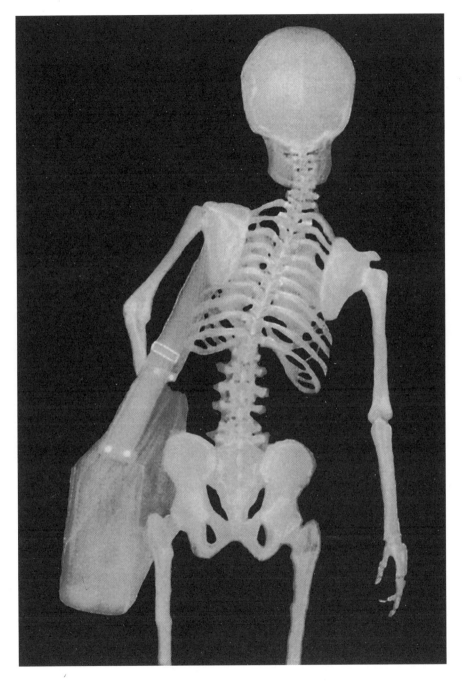

16: Carrying a heavy school bag on one shoulder can put huge pressures on the spine, as is clearly revealed in this X-ray image. This pressure can sow the seeds of future health problems.

report was published by the Research Board for the Correlation of Medical Science and Physical Education. It was found that more than 600 boys and 700 girls had flat feet; 238 boys and 377 girls had hammer toes; at least 702 boys and 718 girls had bent or defective toes, and more than 450 boys and 420 girls had overlapping toes. Furthermore, legs of uneven length were found in 114 boys and 109 girls, and 266 boys and 319 girls had either knock knees or were bow legged. Abnormal curvature of the spine was found in 408 boys and 526 girls, and 337 boys and 372 girls were found to have faulty

17: The weight of school bags often exceeds recommended international industrial guidelines for handling of loads by adults, but who enforces or even checks these guidelines when it comes to children?

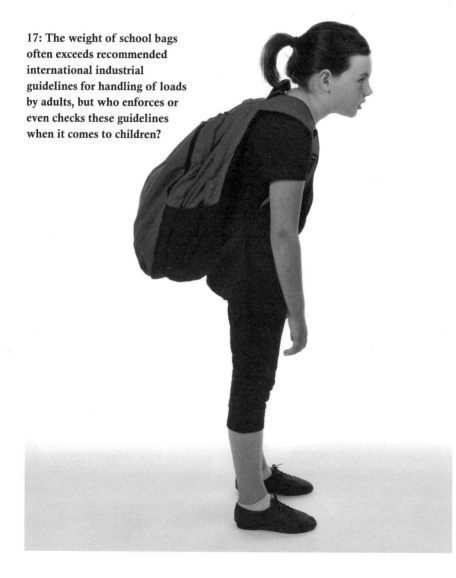

carriage of their heads, i.e. the head was tilted to one side or bent forwards or backwards. Investigators found that most of the defects and deformities tended to become steadily worse as the children got older. All of this added up to a recipe for disaster in later life, and I am sure that today the situation is far worse. All of the above statistics point to the fact that even in the 1950s many children were a long way from the balanced poise, and in my opinion children's posture is far worse today.

In his book *Body Awareness in Action*, Professor Frank Pierce Jones states that two of the most powerful stimuli for producing malposture are a book and a pencil, and it is easy to see that children's posture starts to change within a few years of beginning school. Poor posture in teenagers is now widespread in developed countries, and we are beginning to see it as normal, yet although it is very common it is definitely neither normal nor natural. Many people do not realize that the seeds of ill health are needlessly being sown due to our education system, which has become totally 'results driven'.

A lack of choice

Perhaps all this comes about because, for 11 years of our children's development, we place them in an institution full of 'must', 'have to', 'can't', 'should', 'got to' and 'ought to'. This has the damaging effect of causing children gradually to lose their freedom to choose. If you imprison a bird, at first it will damage itself in its endeavour to escape, every day longing for its freedom to fly unhindered, but if you keep the bird in its cage long enough it will forget that there is anything outside the cage at all. Then, even if you leave the cage door open, the bird will not try to escape – it has resigned itself to being in the cage and has forgotten that there is any other way of existing. In the same way, many children scream, shout and have tantrums during their first days of school, but they 'have to' go, and even the most loving parents will leave their children crying at the school gate regardless of their feelings and parental instincts, because they believe it is 'for their own good'. This can have a detrimental effect on the children, as it may well be the first time they feel abandoned and betrayed, not understanding that the parents themselves really feel that they have no choice.

It is true that, after a few weeks of trauma, children will 'settle down', but what is in fact happening is that they are becoming institutionalized as they learn to conform to what society considers to be the norm. It is not long before many parents can see signs of a change in their children's behaviour as they become more and more withdrawn. By the time these children leave school many years later as young adults they have been conditioned to think and act in certain ways, acquiring fixed prejudices and rigid opinions that often remain with them for the rest of their lives. They feel they must act in a way that fits in with the rest of society, and that if they do not they will be ostracized by their fellow human beings, due to the same prejudices and fears that they have been indoctrinated with during those school years. Yet it is not education that really is the problem, it is the way in which we educate our children. Michael Gelb sums it up in his book, *Body Learning*, when he says:

> This 'disconnected' approach is also evident in our educational system which over-emphasises examination results at the expense of real learning. Our children are fed vast quantities of discrete and often unrelated information which they must parrot back on demand. They are drilled and judged on their performance in a series of disconnected topics. Physical education is usually seen as just another 'subject', quite separate and not as important as the traditional three R's. Indeed the very term 'physical education' suggests the belief that the mind and body can be educated separately.

If education were enjoyable for children, then their posture would reflect that enjoyment and in my view they would not only learn far more quickly, but also learn far more. In fact, children up to the age of five learn a huge amount; most of it is through play without the fear of failure. They learn to stand, walk and talk, and they learn all this in a very effective way, which is generally by copying. Unfortunately, the school system that has evolved over the past century does not take into account how children learn best.

The constant pressure to perform under stressful conditions, whether it is applied at school or later on at work, is one of the primary causes of our degenerating quality of life and ultimately of the stress from which so many of us suffer. A great many people feel that something is missing from their lives, yet because everyone else is in the same position they do not know

18: Long hours bent over a desk can be one of the major causes of poor posture. It can adversely affect breathing and overall wellbeing.

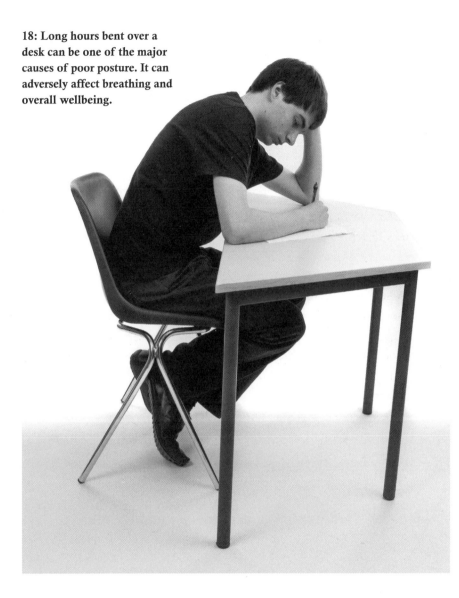

where to turn for advice on increasing their enjoyment of life, and many just end up trying harder and harder, which is exactly the opposite of what they really need to do. Practically every report I brought home from school said, 'Must make more effort' or 'Could try harder', and this is what many people believe life is all about. We make a bigger and bigger effort, yet we end up being further away from the peace and contentment that we long for. In this stressful process we become so anxious that the small pockets of happiness we do experience become less and less frequent. Life is in reality full of pleasure, if we could just stop long enough to appreciate the here and now, rather than hoping that things will get better in the future.

Alexander's view

Alexander was also a firm believer that our education system did not address the real needs of our children, and as a result in 1924 he and his assistants opened a school for children in London. Irene Tasker, a teacher trained by Maria Montessori and also an Alexander teacher, ran what came to be known as 'The Little School', which incorporated teaching children the principles of the Alexander Technique as part of the curriculum. This school offered a completely different approach to education and did not over-stimulate the children's nervous systems, avoiding any over-stimulation of the

" I recommend the Alexander treatment as an extremely sophisticated form of rehabilitation, or rather redeployment, of the entire muscular equipment, and through that of many other organs. Compared with this, many types of physiotherapy which are now in general use look surprisingly crude and restricted in their effect, and sometimes even harmful to the rest of the body.

His [Alexander's] procedure and conclusions meet all the requirements of the strictest scientific method. It [Alexander's technique] bears the same relation to education that education itself bears to all other human activities. "

Dr Alexander Leeper, in a report to the Australian Federal Government's Schools and Registration Board

fear reflexes. The way in which children were taught always took precedence over how much they were taught. This led to calmer emotions and a more open way of learning. In *Constructive Conscious Control of the Individual*, Alexander wrote:

> It occurs to very few parents to consider whether, in this process of 'education' the child's fear reflexes will not be unduly and harmfully excited by the injunction that it must always try to 'be right', indeed, that it is almost a disgrace to be wrong; that the teachers concerned do not even know how to prevent the child from acquiring the very worst psycho-physical use of itself whilst standing or sitting at its desk or table, pondering over its lessons, or performing its other duties.

The habits formed in the school years tend to surface when we later, as adults, try to learn a new subject. The fear of being wrong can develop into a very harmful habit and can really hold us back from learning new subjects, because, of course, in practice, learning anything new always involves making mistakes. John Dewey, the famous philosopher and educator, who was a staunch supporter of Alexander's work, was convinced that people learn far more from making mistakes than from trying to be right. If we have a fear of making mistakes, we tend to hold our breath and assume a harmful posture, as we overexert ourselves, in the same way we did as children while learning to read and write. As adults, we often take these harmful habits into everything that we do and they can affect the way we live our lives, as well as our health.

Recently, neuroscientists have realized that our brain has a quality of what they call 'competitive plasticity'. This simply means that any area in the brain can change its function when required and that the neurological brain map is not static, but can alter to suit the needs of the person. If an area is not used for any given length of time, it will be taken over and used by another of the body's functions. In his book, *The Brain That Changes Itself*, Dr Norman Doidge writes:

> Competitive plasticity also explains why our bad habits are so difficult to break or unlearn. Most of us think of the brain as

a container and learning as putting something in it. When we try to break a bad habit, it takes over the brain map and each time we repeat it, it claims more control of the map and prevents the use of that space for good habit. That is why unlearning is often a lot harder than learning, and why early childhood education is so important – it's best to get it right early before the 'bad habits' get a competitive advantage.

Back in the 1920s, Alexander did not know about modern neuroscience, but he did realize that the prevention of bad habits was far preferable to trying to unlearn them. He also realized that in order to unlearn an undesirable habit, one has to say 'no' to it many times in order for the brain to learn a new way, and this is why he required his students to have lessons daily so that the pupil did not have time to fall back into their old ways of thinking and moving.

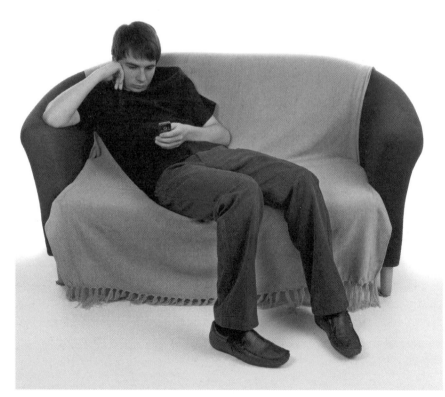

19: Eventually, the bent posture we adopt from working at a school desk for over 15,000 hours becomes a strong habit, which you can easily see in most teenagers.

" Alexander students rid themselves of bad postural
  habits and are helped to reach with their bodies and
  minds an enviable degree of freedom of
  expression. "

Michael Langham, Director, The Juilliard School, New York, USA

John Taylor Gatto, an American teacher and winner of the Teacher of the Year Award three years running, had these strong words to say about the state of education in his article 'Confessions of a Teacher' (published in *Resurgence* magazine in the 1990s): 'By stars and red ticks, smiles and frowns, prizes, honors, and disgraces, I teach you (the child) to surrender your will to the predestined chain of command. Rights may be granted or withheld by any authority without appeal because rights do not exist inside a school, not even the right of free speech, as the Supreme Court has ruled. As a school teacher I intervene in many personal decisions, issuing a pass for those I deem legitimate, or initiating a disciplinary confrontation for behaviour that threatens my control. As individuality is constantly trying to assert itself among children and teenagers, my judgments come thick and fast. Individuality is a contradiction of class theory, a curse to all systems of classification.'

The self-confidence that very young children naturally possess can be maintained only in the absence of stress, confusion, uncertainty and, most of all, the fear of failure. Unfortunately, these are the very forces inflicted upon many children to 'keep them under control'. My aim here is not to blame individual teachers or parents, but rather to reflect on the way in which education has evolved as a whole. Because of our own experiences, we also can behave as our own parents or teachers behaved, unwittingly contributing to the pressure on our children. How frequently do we tell our children how wonderful they are, or how well they are doing? Sadly, we are often far too busy nowadays even to notice. Their 'naughty' behaviour patterns are usually a desperate attempt to get noticed or to relieve boredom.

The way in which we were treated as children has an enormous influence on how we live the rest of our lives, and many of the behaviour patterns that

20: The unnatural and unhealthy bend in the upper spine, which is often caused by working for long hours at the school desk, soon feels 'normal' in every action we do.

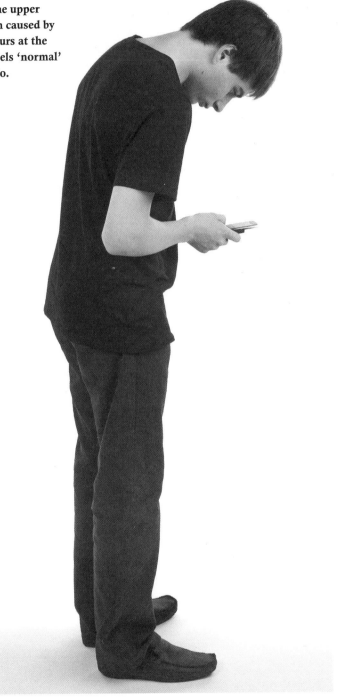

we repeat through our adult lives are formed in early childhood. As children, we learn everything we know from mimicking those around us, and at first we do not even judge the actions that we are copying. The habits acquired then often only emerge 20 or 30 years later, when we have children of our own. Children are not born with fixed opinions or prejudices; these are acquired without question from the environment in which they live. It can be useful to question aspects of our lives to see if we are living as we would choose to, or merely trying to live up to other people's expectations without realizing it.

Although we are not individually to blame for the goal-oriented way that education has developed, we do have a responsibility to change it. The best way that we can help children is to stop imposing rigid rights and wrongs, in order to reduce the level of fear that they experience (what Alexander called 'unduly excited fear reflexes'). If we can give them confidence by encouraging them, rather than promoting fear of ridicule and punishment for getting things wrong, we will be helping them in a fundamental way to improve their wellbeing, which in turn will beneficially affect their posture. If we can teach our children in a way that enhances their self-esteem, they will not only learn more, but also lead more harmonious and creative lives.

Another consideration in all this is that of speed. Not only do we want our children to have a great deal of knowledge about as much as possible, we also want them to put it down on paper as fast as possible. If you remember the time when you were sitting your own exams, you were probably given so little time to complete the paper that you felt rushed from the moment you sat down. This again excites what Alexander called 'the fear reflexes' and in turn affects posture. This pressure to rush many of our activities is such an important point that I have dedicated the whole of the next chapter to it.

CHAPTER 7

The Secret Key to Good Posture

What lies behind us and what lies before us are tiny matters compared to what lies within us.

Ralph Waldo Emerson

We are living in the 'speed age' where we are surrounded by a vast range of inventions that have been designed to save us time. These include the car, the computer, the dishwasher, the vacuum cleaner, the washing machine, the telephone, electric heaters, electric tools... the list is a long one. In fact, during the 1950s in the USA people were getting very concerned about what they were going to do to with all their spare time, now that they had so many time-saving devices! The only problem is that here we are, a few decades later, and a great many people feel that they have less time than before. Posture and time are very much connected, as can be seen in common expressions such as being 'pressed for time', 'pushed for time' 'under pressure of time', or 'moving at breakneck speed'. This feeling that we have too little time causes harmful tension throughout the body. The old adage that 'there is never enough time to do a job properly, but there is always time to go back and correct the mistakes' makes the point that there really was enough time in the first place. Lack of time is more of a feeling or a thought than a reality. As young children we felt we had all the time in the world, and we were firmly rooted in the present moment. The summer months seemed endless, as did the time from one Christmas to another. Having little or no concept of time, young children do not run because they feel late – they run because they enjoy running. This lack of awareness of time is reflected in graceful posture and movements. As we get older, however, time restraints put on us by school or work commitments cause us to become more and more concerned about the consequences of being late, and we are encouraged to develop over-concern for the future, thus being less and less engaged in the present moment. Our lives as adults are commonly filled with appointments for specific times, and if we are late we feel that there may be trouble, even if we are simply meeting a friend for coffee.

Life is not an emergency

Jean Liedloff, an American psychologist who spent two and a half years in the South American jungle with South American Indians, saw that they had little or no concept of time. In her book *The Continuum Concept* she relates that she saw that the indigenous people were in no rush to finish one task so that they could get on to the next thing. They were happy in the present moment focusing on whatever tasks they were doing, and they were not thinking ahead to the future or having regrets about their past actions. As a result, she noticed, they were far happier and more contented than people in developed countries. They laughed rather than cursed when things went wrong, and were far more alert, aware and connected to the things around them. Liedloff's experience challenged radically her Western preconceptions of how we should live and led her to a very different view of human nature.

We are generally taught, implicitly or explicitly, that doing things quickly is far better than doing things well. Many of us feel that every job we undertake has to be done quickly, and yet this takes the enjoyment out of the work. One consequence of this is that many people stop enjoying their work, and this only makes matters worse, because it encourages them to rush it even more to get the task over with. Alexander believed that the human race was becoming increasingly goal-oriented, and that this affects our posture in a detrimental way; in fact, in *The Use of the Self* he says that when we are living a life dominated by speed, we are on 'the royal road to the physical and mental derangement of mankind'. Have a look outside any school after the morning bell has rung, or an office after work begins. You will see children, parents and workers rushing to get to their destination. Typically their shoulders will be hunched up and forward, their heads will be pulled back and down onto their spines and their backs will be arched. If this is repeated every day, these postural deformities become habits and eventually become fixed within the body. Ram Dass (aka Dr Richard Alpert), an American spiritual teacher who spent a great deal of time in India, often said that one of the most important things people in the West need to learn is that 'life is not an emergency'. Another thought-provoking saying is: 'Man says: "Quickly, quickly, hurry up. Time is passing away", but Time says: "It is not me that passes away, it is man!" If you spend some time thinking about it, it may change your perspective on life.

So a vital step in improving posture is to begin to give ourselves more time in everything we do. Realizing that life is not one long emergency really helps to improve posture. This may sound simple but it is difficult to practise when we have lifelong habits of rushing around. When I first moved to Ireland in the mid- 1990s, to make conversation I used to ask people what they did for a living. I nearly always got the same answer – 'As little as possible!' – and you could see this in the way they took their time and enjoyed their various tasks. To me this is actually what the Alexander Technique sets out to achieve: going about our activities with as little tension as needed. In the late 1990s, Ireland enjoyed a period of unprecedented economic growth and prosperity (the so-called 'Celtic Tiger'), and people weren't giving the same answer any more, as everyone started to do as much as they possibly could. The relaxed way of life soon became a thing of the past as Ireland quickly caught up with the ways of other modern developed countries.

The habit of rushing

The habit of rushing from one thing to the next is a problem that affects us physically, mentally, emotionally and spiritually. It can cause anxiety, which in extreme cases may permeate our whole existence until life feels hardly worth living. It affects us physically in such a way that our whole system is constantly on 'red alert', ageing us before our time. It may even cause or exacerbate stress-related illnesses such as hypertension, strokes and heart problems, which are life-threatening.

Feeling that we do not have enough time affects us mentally by over-stimulating the mind, eventually causing mental blocks, an over-active mind, which gives us little or no control over persistent unwanted thoughts, and

" It gives us all the things we have been looking for in a system of physical education: relief from strain due to maladjustment, and consequent improvement in physical and mental health, increased consciousness of the physical means employed to gain the ends proposed by the will and, along with this, a general heightening of consciousness on all levels...We cannot ask more from any system of physical education; nor, if we seriously desire to alter human beings in a desirable direction, can we ask any less. "

Aldous Huxley, writer

endless worry for no reason. It affects us emotionally because it can cause us to lose control of our anger and react irrationally, which eventually can damage relationships with family or friends. It can affect us spiritually, because it prevents us from being in contact with the peace and tranquillity that should be the very essence and foundation of our life. Stress prevents us from 'being human' in the truest sense of the word and turns us into 'doing machines', which in time will start to break us down.

At first, we may actively enjoy the buzz of the adrenalin as it rushes around the body when we take on an exciting new challenge, but sustained over the long term stress can rob us of everything that is important. It can take away our good health and replace it with an aching head or back, or one of a wide range of other stress-related disorders. We can forget how to relax. It can destroy our personal relationships and, as a result, cause extreme emotional anguish. How often do we really pause for even a moment to see whether the path we have taken in life is actually making us more satisfied, fulfilled and contented? Since happiness is the natural antidote to stress, maybe we first need to take a good hard look at the ways in which we try to become happy and find out why it is that, in our endeavour to achieve this goal, we can end up feeling more stressed than ever. We could then perhaps find new ways that may be more successful that involve taking our time. There is an interesting saying in *The Talmud* that says, 'Whoever forces time is pushed back by time; whoever yields to time finds time on his side.' Other proverbs and sayings include:

No time like the present

Look before you leap

More haste, less speed

All good things come to those who wait

Rome was not built in a day

Fools rush in where angels fear to tread

Second thoughts are best

Good and quickly seldom meet

The first steps in changing habits

The first thing to do is to notice how you feel when you are in a hurry. Notice the position of your head and shoulders. See if you can feel tension in other parts of your body, for example your back, legs, arms and even your jaw. Ask yourself how important is it that you get to your destination as quickly as possible. You may realize that there is actually no hurry and that you are rushing out of habit. It is important to differentiate between doing things quickly and rushing our movements; there is nothing wrong about doing things quickly, it is constant hurrying that harms us.

Inhibition

As we saw in Chapter 2, Alexander realized that the only way he could prevent his habit was to inhibit the immediate reaction to a stimulus that encouraged or caused a habit. Inhibition is one of the two parts of the Alexander Technique (the other being direction), and without it we do not have a chance to change our behaviour. It is not easy to inhibit a reaction that has become so familiar, yet inhibit we must if we want change in our lives. After all, to quote Anthony Robbins, 'If you do what you've always done, you'll get what you've always gotten.' It may be that the rushing around feels so right and natural to us that when we give ourselves more time it may well feel like something is wrong. The rushing habit needs to be replaced by a different way of being, and that is bound to feel strange or alien for a while, but that is the nature of changing habits. When we are able to stop that reaction and choose a different response to the many demands that are placed on us, we will feel calmer and more able to cope with life.

In recent times, the word *inhibition* has come to mean the suppression of feelings or the inability to be spontaneous, but this is mainly because the famous psychiatrist Sigmund Freud used the term in this particular context. The dictionary definition of inhibition is: 'The restraint of direct expression of an instinct'. If this restraint stems from fear and is unconscious, then it could be seen as involving an unhealthy form of suppression and would therefore have a negative connotation. However, Alexander used the term to mean 'deliberately refraining from one's automatic habitual reaction in order to make a more conscious decision', which can have very beneficial results. Dr Jacob Bronowski, author of *The Ascent of Man*, went so far as to say: 'We are nature's unique experiment to make the rational intelligence prove sounder than the reflex. Success or failure of this experiment depends on the basic human ability to impose a delay between the stimulus and the response.' This states exactly what Alexander was writing about 50 years before. In his book, *Body Awareness in Action*, Professor Frank Pierce Jones describes inhibition as: 'the fundamental process, conscious or unconscious, by which the integrity of the organism is maintained while a particular response is being carried out, or not carried out, as the case may be. It is the failure of inhibition that more than anything else is responsible for the dangerous state of the world. Restoring inhibition so that it can perform its integrative function on a conscious level should be the primary aim of education.'

A good example of inhibition can be seen by observing the domestic cat chasing its prey. It pauses before springing forward to ensure the best chance of success. And just notice the posture of a cat! Applying inhibition does not mean that we cannot move quickly when we wish – cats move very quickly when they want to, but they are never in a hurry to get the next job done. Through this process of consciously choosing a different way of reacting, we can start to claim back our lives and live in a way that we choose, and our posture will reflect this change.

Inhibition also has another important function: it helps us engage in a process of 'unlearning'. We were not born with poor posture (or poor use of ourselves): this is a learnt behaviour and as a result needs to be 'unlearnt'. Inhibition gives us a chance to prevent our stereotyped patterns of movement; and if we can prevent our harmful habits, the right way of moving will return. In other words, if we have a habit of pulling our head back onto our spine, all we have to do is prevent this habit and the right movement will manifest. It is not a question of finding the right posture or correct way of standing, sitting or moving – that is already within us. A postural habit, like any other habit, is difficult to break initially and will take perseverance. This is because our habits by their very nature are self-sustaining. Going back to *The Brain That Changes Itself*, Dr Norman Doidge writes: 'Different chemistries are involved in learning than in unlearning. When we learn something new, neurons fire together and wire together, and a chemical process occurs at the neuronal level called "long-term potentiation" or LTP, which strengthens connections between the neurons. When the brain unlearns associations and disconnects neurons, another chemical process occurs, called "long-term depression", or LTD (which has nothing to do with a depressed mood state). Unlearning and weakening connections between neurons is just a plastic process, and just as important as learning and strengthening them. If we only strengthened connections, our neuronal networks would get saturated. Evidence suggests that unlearning existing memories is necessary to make room for new memories in our networks.' So when you inhibit your habitual response, you are in effect making room for something new to take place; and if you repeat the process many times, eventually the new improved way of moving will then feel normal to you.

“ The Alexander Technique transformed my life.
It is the result of an acknowledged genius. I would
recommend it to anyone. ”

Tony Buzan, author of *Use Your Head* and creator of Mind Mapping

Give yourself time

Your life takes place only in the here and now. When rushing towards some future task, we are missing life completely. Have you ever wondered why, when you were a child, the summer days seemed endless, yet now time passes so quickly? The reason is that we are no longer in the present: we are too busy thinking of the past and future. But nothing ever happens in the future or the past, everything happens in the present moment. The Alexander Technique is a practical way of helping to keep our consciousness in the here and now. If you find it hard not to be overly concerned about the future, it might be helpful to realize that the way we live our lives in the present moment is actually what shapes our future. Giving ourselves time is the best present we can give ourselves, yet in reality we are really only claiming what is rightfully ours in the first place. There are many old sayings that speak of the benefits of taking our time; just recently I came across this Old Irish saying, which is worth remembering:

> Take time to work – it is the price of success.
>
> Take time to meditate – it is the source of power.
>
> Take time to play – it is the secret of perpetual youth.
>
> Take time to read – it is the way to knowledge.
>
> Take time to be friendly – it is the road to happiness.
>
> Take time to laugh – it is the music of the soul.
>
> Take time to love and be loved.

Some time ago, a woman came to see me suffering from stress. She felt that her whole life was one big rush, and she used to come to nearly every lesson with her head retracted backwards and her shoulders nearly touching her ears. After each lesson she felt much more relaxed and her posture had greatly improved, yet when she came back the following week, the effects of the Alexander lesson has almost completely worn off. At the beginning of most lessons, she would practically run into the room, out of breath, and would then spend half of the time recovering from her rushing habit. After several lessons she came in one day a completely different person. She walked up the stairs with her shoulders relaxed and her head balanced freely on the spine. I remarked on the difference and asked her why she thought this dramatic change had happened at that time. She told me that she had just celebrated her birthday, and her family had become so exasperated with her stressed behaviour that they had brought her a new watch – a special one. On this watch there was no minute hand, and instead of the usual numbers printed around the clock face, each hour was marked 'one-ish', 'two-ish', 'three-ish' and so on. So she no longer knew the precise time, and therefore never knew when she was late or when she was early, and this had had a profound effect on her life (I should point out that she was never very late!).

So, the key to good posture is really to take *your* time as you go about your daily activities, and pause for a moment and consider how to perform a certain task even if that task is simply sitting down or standing up. Just try it for a day and you will find that this would go a long way to not only improving your posture, but also revolutionizing the way you live.

CHAPTER 8

The Effects of Furniture on Posture

The rise in back problems over the last century correlates directly with the increasing number of hours we spend seated.

Professor Galen Cranz, author of *The Chair*

While it is true that the Alexander Technique is principally concerned with improving the way we use ourselves by eradicating detrimental habits that affect our posture, I personally think it is also of great benefit to find out how and why many of these habits originated, so that we can avoid the same problems in the future – and what we sit on affects the way we sit. If some of our postural problems are caused or exacerbated by environmental factors that encourage poor posture, it would obviously be beneficial if we can start to change these, as well as ourselves. In my opinion, one of the major external causes of poor posture is badly designed furniture, and by using chairs that are 'human friendly' we will stand a much better chance of maintaining good posture.

It is interesting to observe that back pain and neck problems have reached epidemic proportions in all countries where sitting on chairs has become the norm, and chairs and desks are the most common ergonomic factors that encourage poor posture. Many of us spend as much as 75 per cent of our waking lives sitting on chairs: we sit to eat, we sit at the computer and we sit in the car or on a train or bus when travelling to work and in our homes when relaxing. In the USA, they even have drive-through movies, banks, churches, takeaways and supermarkets. It is sometimes hard to know where it is all going to end – perhaps one day there will be drive-through dentists and doctors as well! But the less we stand and walk, the less we like standing and walking: it becomes a vicious circle. In this chapter, we will analyse if what we are sitting on is in harmony with how the body is designed to sit.

Chairs

Many people do not realize that the chairs they use can actually mould the form of the human body and can so severely affect posture that I often refer to them as 'weapons of mass destruction'. Driving for long distances in badly designed car seats can practically cripple us, so by the end of the journey we can barely straighten up afterwards. I thought it would be interesting to find out who designs these kind of seats, which are not only uncomfortable but can actually be harmful when used for long periods, and to find out why they are designed in this way. Some years ago I was invited to Middlesex University in the UK to talk about the Alexander Technique to students in their final year of a degree course in furniture design. Before I began my lecture, I asked the students what is the first thing that they think about before they design a chair. Nearly all of them gave me the same answer: 'Colour!' I was a little surprised because I had expected them to be thinking of something more technical like the height or how the chair supported the human frame. I was intrigued by their answer and wanted to know more. 'Why colour?' I asked them. 'It's obvious', they said. 'If you designed the best chair in the world, but covered it with lime green material, nobody would buy it.' And then it dawned on me that most furniture designers are putting a great deal of emphasis on whether the chair *looks* aesthetically pleasing but are paying little attention to designing for the human being who is going to use the furniture. A chair that has lots of inviting curves may initially feel comfortable as we sink into it, but the same chair may offer inadequate support and in the long term put unnecessary strains and stresses on the body.

Let's analyse the process that young children typically go through when they start to sit for longer and longer periods, to see if there is something to be learnt from it. While at school, most of us sit for over 15,000 hours, which is a huge amount of time, especially if the chair design is putting unnecessary strain on the muscles and joints. It is simply not natural to sit for prolonged periods, no matter how good the chair is, because as we have already mentioned, the body is primarily designed for movement rather than keeping still.

The decline of upright posture

As soon as children go to school at the age of four or five, they are forced to sit in a chair – they have no choice. The teacher, who often has around 30 children to cope with, cannot keep his or her eye on all the children if they are moving freely around the classroom. Since the teacher's main responsibility is for the safety of all these children, he or she will usually insist that they remain in their chairs for most of the day. The children do not like sitting down for very long, as they find the chair itself is very uncomfortable

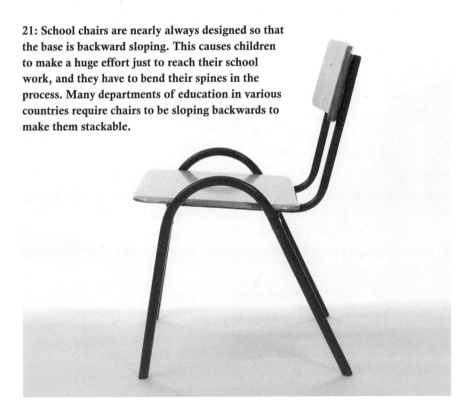

21: School chairs are nearly always designed so that the base is backward sloping. This causes children to make a huge effort just to reach their school work, and they have to bend their spines in the process. Many departments of education in various countries require chairs to be sloping backwards to make them stackable.

and is not suited to their natural posture. The main reason for the discomfort is that the *horizontal* part of the chair, which takes most of the weight of the body, is *sloping backwards*. Most school chairs are designed in this way because it allows them to be stacked without the danger of falling over, and while that may be more convenient for the cleaners, it is a disaster for the children's natural upright posture.

When children sit on this kind of backward-sloping furniture, which is the norm in many schools, they have no option but to tense many of their muscles in order to maintain an upright posture. I believe that this tension represents the beginning of the numerous musculoskeletal and respiratory problems that we see in our culture today. The children feel uncomfortable, and within minutes they will try to get up and move around the classroom. In most cases, they are immediately instructed to sit down again.

Children have a natural ingenuity and intelligence when it comes to posture and body awareness, and so their next instinctive strategy is to try to counteract the 'falling backwards' movement produced by the chair by tilting themselves forwards, raising the back legs of the chair off the floor as they do this. This is an intelligent strategy because it corrects the backward slope of the chair seat, making it level or slightly forward-sloping, and this helps the children to maintain an aligned, upright posture with much less effort. Instead of being curious as to why so many children are tilting their chairs forwards, however, we just tell them exactly what we were told ourselves: 'Don't tip the chairs – you will break them!' Of course, the teacher is mindful of the danger that someone could trip over the back legs, or that the children might tilt too far, fall forward and hurt themselves, but it is interesting to note that it is usually the possible damage to the chair that is given as the reason to stop a child from doing this. The damage to the child's posture is not even considered or noticed at any stage.

The children still do not give up; they then often develop other techniques to counter the effects of the backward slope, such as sitting on a foot, which also has the effect of raising the pelvis. This is just another way of enabling them to pivot on the sitting bones, again keeping an aligned and healthy spine; however, it is often actively discouraged in case the blood flow to the leg is restricted.

Once they have been prevented from doing what comes naturally to them, eventually the children have to give up, and they learn to endure sitting on

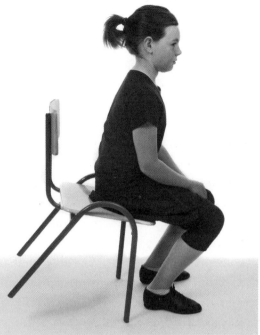

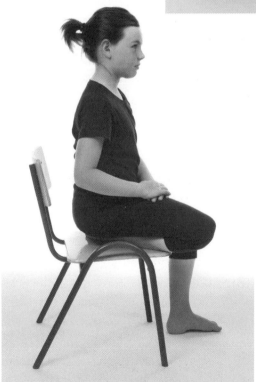

22: At first children alter the angle of the base by tipping the chair forward, which in effect makes the chair into a forward-sloping chair.

23: If children are not allowed to tip the chair forward, they often resort to sitting on one leg, which can affect the blood flow down the leg.

backward-sloping chairs for literally thousands and thousands of hours while at school. Sooner or later most, if not all, of them, slowly but surely begin to slump as their back muscles become more and more fatigued. To make matters worse, consider that the children also have to bend over their desks for a large proportion of this time in order to read and write. Since it is very difficult for them to use their hip joints efficiently while sitting on backward-sloping chairs, and the pelvis itself is already rotating backwards, the only option left open to them is to bend their upper back and necks forward, often quite severely. Over time this way of sitting becomes a habit, and many teenagers have a very bent posture even when they are not working at a desk, which can cause unnecessary wear and tear on the vertebrae and discs, thus sowing the seeds of future spinal and back problems.

In effect, what we are doing is this: first we ruin children's posture by making them sit on badly designed furniture and then, in our ignorance, we chastise the children for slumping. It is pure madness! As their posture begins to deteriorate over the years, they are told to 'sit up straight' and 'put your shoulders back', but the only way to do this is to over-arch the lumbar spine and contract many of the powerful back muscles, which are already tense. Worse still, the children then begin to think that this is the way they ought to sit. Unfortunately, this rigid posture becomes fixed within the body and can often remain with them for the rest of their days, causing their muscles and joints to become progressively stiffer or more painful as time goes on. It really is a catalogue of disasters, but fortunately for us the solution to this problem is a simple one.

Before we can start to improve sitting, we need to understand a little about the design of the human frame. The bones that we sit on are often

" The Alexander Technique makes a real difference to my often tense and busy life. Its thoughtful approach has made me calmer, improved my concentration and given me a clearer sense of my own wellbeing. I am grateful for it. "

Joan Bakewell, journalist, writer and TV presenter

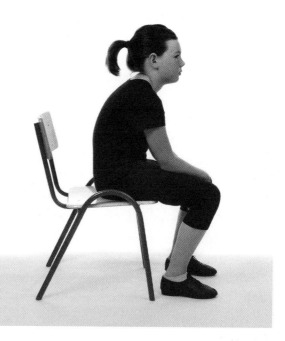

24: Even without bending over their desks, children become slumped when sitting on backward slopng furniture... and so do adults.

25: Adding a <u>firm</u> wedge-shaped cushion to a backward-sloping chair can dramatically help to maintain good posture and beneficial breathing habits.

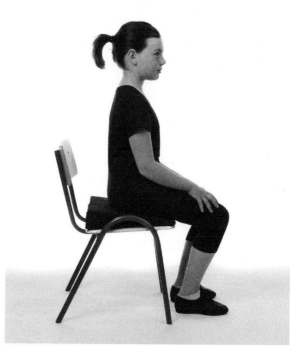

referred to as the 'sitting bones' (or *ischial tuberosities*) but are, in fact, the lowest part of the pelvis. If you look at the image of the pelvis on page 113, you will notice that these bones are rounded, and it is not difficult to see that if you put this obviously rounded surface on the backward-sloping base of a chair, gravity will cause it to rock backwards. (If you place a marble or golf ball on a typical backward-sloping chair or car seat, you will see what I mean.) This backward and downward force is exerted on the sitting bones, yet it is these bones that children need to use in order to pivot themselves forward while reading and writing at a desk. Once they find they are unable to rock forward on the sitting bones (because it is very difficult to rock uphill), they will unconsciously find another way to reach the desk, and this usually involves actually bending their spine, which soon causes a misalignment of the entire spine. This bent back eventually becomes a permanent habit, as can be seen in so many teenagers when they sit, stand and walk – even when there is no need. As you can see on page 91, when a child is sitting on a level base or with a small forward slope, her back is very straight (photo 25), yet the same child distorts her back when sitting on a chair that slopes backwards (photo 24).

Since many of us have been through this same process in our own childhood, it is hardly surprising that there are millions of people at this very moment suffering with lower back pain. I am personally convinced that school furniture and the tense postures we were told to hold as children have contributed directly to the phenomenal rise in back and neck pain in recent years. This has been backed up by a detailed report by the National Back Pain Association UK, published in October 2005, which stated:

> Sustained poor posture, which is probably the key environmental cause of back pain in children and adolescents, results from a combination of factors, the most significant of these seems to be the inappropriate furniture at school.

Elizabeth Langford sums up the situation very well in her book, *Mind and Muscle*, when she writes: 'No amount of "physical education" will undo the damage done to schoolchildren condemned to spend hours of every day sitting on such chairs. Good chairs can never guarantee good sitting, but it is scandalous that children, forced to use chairs on which it is impossible to sit

The cycle of discomfort

When we use a chair whose base slopes backwards, we are actively encouraged to lean backwards and seek support from the back of the chair. This initiates a backward and downward force. The heavier we are, or the greater degree of habitual muscular tension there is in the body, the greater that force will be. The downward force pushes the base of the pelvis forward and eventually we find ourselves sitting with our weight behind the tailbone rather than on the sitting bones, which have been tilted backwards. This, in turn, encourages the spine to adopt a 'C'-shaped slouch, causing compression in the lungs and other internal organs and strain on the ribs and diaphragm and all the intervertebral discs in the lumbar spine. After a short time, we find this position uncomfortable, so we try to sit up straight by over-arching the lumbar area. Soon we find this position tiring and again seek support from the back of the chair and the whole cycle starts all over again.

properly, are thus moulded for a future of poor co-ordination, back pain, and other health problems.'

These days the problem can start even earlier than school, because now most children's pushchairs and car seats are also following this trend and sloping backwards. In fact, the base of nearly every car seat, chair and sofa slopes backwards, and nowadays some even have the added problem of a firm 'lumbar support' pushing into the lower back at the same time. It is hardly surprising that many people have acute back pain after a long drive or when sitting in such a chair for a long time.

As has been thoroughly established by now, back pain is a serious problem in our society today. However, fortunately the solution for correcting chairs is very simple. To solve the problem, all you need to do is alter the base of the chair so it is no longer sloping backwards. This can easily be achieved by using a wedge-shaped cushion. You can also achieve the same effect by taking two books, about 5cm (2in) thick (old telephone books are ideal), and placing one under each of the back legs of the chair. This will make the base of the chair flat or sloping slightly forwards, which will encourage you to pivot on your sitting bones when leaning forwards. Obviously the books are

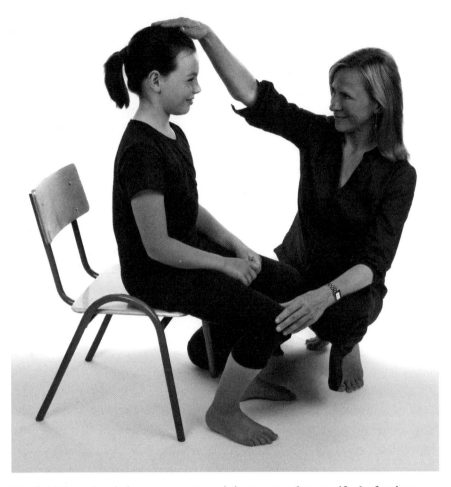

26: If children already have poor posture, it is not enough to rectify the furniture. They will need to have some Alexander lessons to unlearn their bad postural habits.

not practical for everyday use, but the wedges can be obtained from most back shops. Make sure that the wedge you buy is made from good quality hard foam. Those made from softer foam may be cheaper, but they are much less effective.

It is important to use the wedge-shaped cushion for only one hour on the first day and then gradually build up the amount of time you spend sitting on it. This allows time for your muscles to get used to a new and improved way of sitting. After about three to four weeks, you will be able to sit on the cushion comfortably for as long as you like. It is also important to get up and move at least once an hour, because even with the cushion long periods of sitting, on even the best chairs, can still be detrimental. Even better, if you buy a chair that is fully adjustable, you can adjust the angle of the base so you can have it in different positions to suit the task you are doing. Details of websites where you can get good-quality wedges and adjustable chairs can be found on page 179. It is important to note that wedges and forward-sloping chairs are to be used only while you are sitting in activity and not particularly when you are resting. The times when it is most helpful to use the wedge cushion is when you need to lean forward for some reason, such as when writing, working at a computer, eating a meal or driving.

Another important factor when considering the design of chairs is height. It is often the case that the height of a chair is virtually the same for all chairs, yet human beings are very different in size. According to the *Guinness World Records*, the tallest person in the world is 2.46m (8ft 1in), while the shortest is 0.7m (2ft 5in), so it is also very important that your chair is the correct height for you. A rough rule of thumb is that your chair needs to be a third of your height.

Desks

Desks can be a problem, too. Most desks are also designed to a standard height, so for many people the desk can be too high while for others the same desk can be too low. This can be very problematic during school years, when children are growing at different rates. Your desk should be roughly half your height, but if you change the height of your desk or chair, do allow a little time to get used to the new way of working.

In the past, many school desks used to slope forwards (i.e. they were higher at the back than at the front), like many of the writing desks that you can still buy today, but in recent times most desks have become flat. Writing at a flat desk is harder work because the person has to bend further to write, and this causes more strain. So, with the combination of backward-sloping chairs and flat desks, we now have to bend our spines forwards far more than ever before. Once again, though, the solution is easy, as you can buy or make a small sloping writing platform to put on the desk. If the surface that you are writing on is sloping towards you and the chair is also sloping forwards (as in photo 28), you will find that the angle you have to bend is

27: Children contort their bodies in reaction to badly designed classroom furniture – a familiar scene in a great many classrooms today.

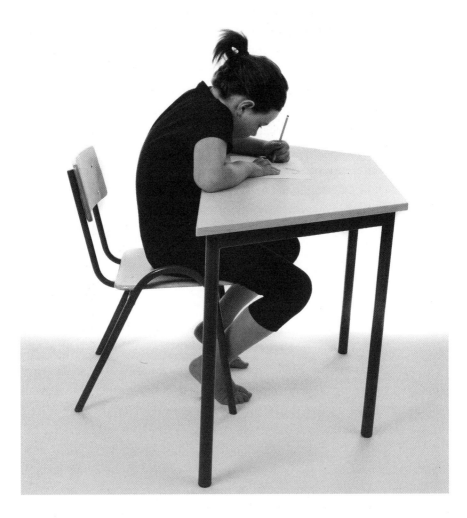

greatly reduced and therefore will put much less pressure on the muscles, bones and joints. It may well save you a lot of time and trouble if you get an Alexander teacher to show you how to achieve the optimum posture while sitting in this new way rather than trying to work it out on your own.

If you are one of those millions of people who spend many hours a day working at a desk, you will find these small, simple changes invaluable in

28: With a wedge-shaped cushion, a writing platform and some Alexander lessons, this child is sitting quite differently than in photo 27. Her poise, grace of movement and even her overall behaviour can be transformed.

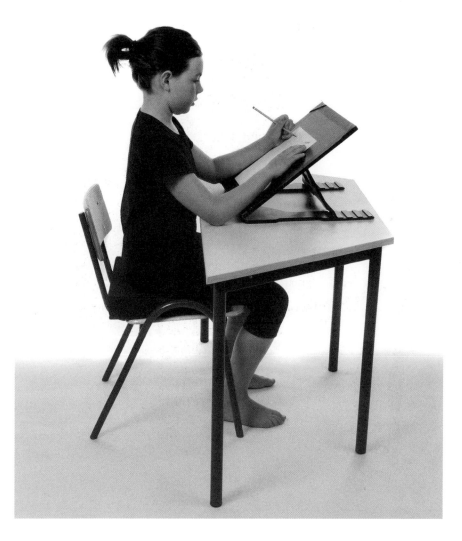

helping you to maintain a healthy posture once you have changed your detrimental habits. So, if we apply the Alexander Technique to change the way we use ourselves, and at the same time we alter our chairs and desks to suit us better, this combined strategy can be very empowering for those whose physical pain is exacerbated by prolonged sitting.

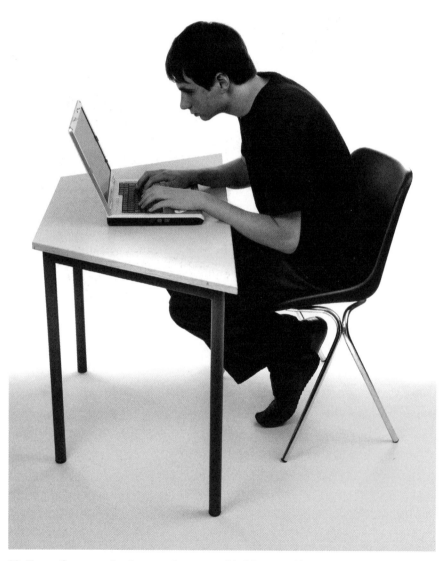

29: Even after our school years, the postural habits prevail as we continue to sit in our habitual way. Without awareness of these habits they often become more and more ingrained as we become older.

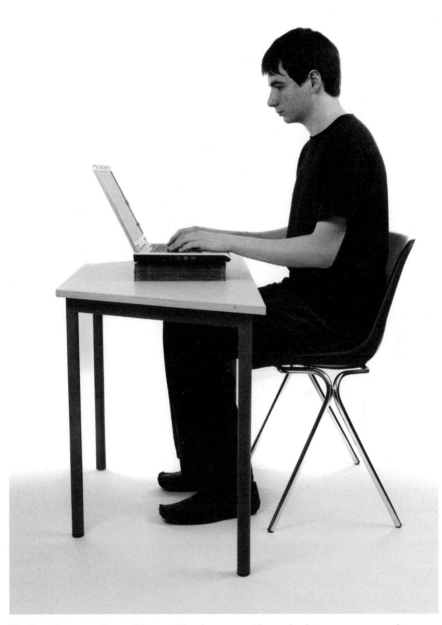

30: By using a wedge cushion and having some Alexander lessons, we can relearn how to sit, stand and move with an overall improved use of ourselves. Raising the computer screen may also encourage an upright posture.

CHAPTER 9

The Hidden Obstacle
to Improving Posture

Everyone wants to be right, but no one stops to consider
if their idea of right is right. When people are wrong,
the thing that is right is bound to be wrong to them.

F Matthias Alexander

The main obstacle that gets in the way of posture improvement is what Alexander called 'faulty sensory appreciation', and this must be taken into account when we try to improve the way we use ourselves. Faulty sensory appreciation simply means that the feedback mechanisms that tell us where we are in space are defective and are often relaying unreliable information. In other words, although we are often absolutely convinced that we have a particular posture or have a certain way of moving, the reality is that we may well be doing something totally different to what we think. It is not until we catch sight of our reflection in a mirror or shop window that we realize how different our posture is from the way we think it is, as this slightly adapted poem by Irish philosopher Edmund Burke (1729–97) illustrates:

I look in the mirror
And what do I see?
A strange looking person
That cannot be me.

For I am much taller
And not nearly so fat
As that man in the mirror
I am looking at.

Oh, where are the mirrors
That I used to know
Like the ones which were
Made thirty years ago?

Now all things have changed
And I'm sure you'll agree
Mirrors are not as good
As they used to be.

So never be concerned,
If stoops appear
For one thing I've learned
Which is very clear,

Should your posture
Be less than perfection,
It must be the mirror
That needs correction!!

In *The Use of the Self,* Alexander noted at first:

> how confident I was... that I should be able to put into
> practice any idea that I thought desirable. When I found
> myself unable to do so, I thought that this was merely a
> personal idiosyncrasy, but my teaching experience of the past
> thirty-five years and my observation of people with whom I
> have come into contact in other ways have convinced me
> that this was not an idiosyncrasy, but that most people would
> have done the same in similar circumstances. I was indeed
> suffering from a delusion that is practically universal.

What that means is that unless we realize that our kinaesthetic sense is probably unreliable, we do not stand much chance of improving our posture, because nearly everyone is relying on their feeling to tell them what is correct or incorrect. So the first thing we need to learn is the difference between what we believe we are doing and what we are really doing. Any belief about posture is based on a feeling that is likely to be distorted. A good example of this is when we catch ourselves on video or in a mirror and our image does not match our sense of where we are in space. This kind of unreliable or faulty sensory feeling is very common when it comes to posture, and an example of this that many people experience during Alexander lessons is when they totally believe that they are sitting or standing up straight when in fact it is clear to an observer that they are leaning backwards or to one side.

The six senses

Over 2,000 years ago, Aristotle described the five senses of sight, hearing, smell, taste and touch, which are the ones most people are aware of today, but we also have an internal sense, which even today for the most part goes unmentioned. This internal sense, which we can call the sixth sense, gives us information about balance, posture and coordination and is the result of several body systems working together. In order to achieve balance, we require information from the visual system (eyes), the vestibular system (ears), the body's sense of where it is in space (proprioception) and the internal sense of movement or motion (kinaesthesia). Kinaesthesia is proprioception while moving. This information is received and organized by the brain. If the information or our interpretation of this information is faulty, then we can never really improve our posture as we will constantly be adopting certain positions because they 'feel right' rather than because they are natural.

The kinaesthetic sense

The word *kinaesthetic* is an ancient Greek compound of *cineō* (which means 'motion') and *aesthēsis*, (which means 'sensation'). The kinaesthetic sense uses input receptors from within the muscles and joints; it also sends messages to the brain whenever there is movement. These sensations send impulses along nerves to the brain and thus inform us of any movement that the body is making, even the movements of breathing.

31: Many people are, in fact, leaning back even when they think they are straight. This may be one of the major causes of lower back pain because leaning backwards can put considerable pressure on the lumbar spine.

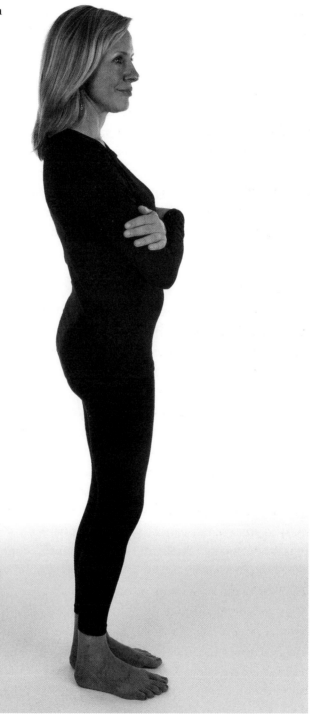

The sense of proprioception

The word *proprioception* comes from two Latin words: *proprius*, meaning 'one's own', and *percepio*, meaning 'to gain, learn, perceive or understand'. It is the sense that informs us of the relative position of parts of the body to each other at any given moment in time. Like the kinaesthetic sense, it is referred to as an internal, or interoceptive, sense, because it is stimulated from within the body itself. This is done via numerous sensory receptors in the internal organs and the inner ear, as well as joint and muscle receptors, all of which are neurologically linked to the brain. The term was coined in 1906 by the English neurophysiologist Charles Sherrington, who received the Nobel Prize in Physiology or Medicine in 1932 for research on the function of the neuron and study of reflex action. Sherrington was also a pupil of Alexander and a staunch supporter of his work.

Faulty sensory awareness

Kinaesthesia and proprioception are often used interchangeably, though the former, strictly speaking, refers to our perception of the relative positions of our limbs and other body parts in space during movement, while the latter is the same thing when we are stationary. They are both extremely important for coordination, balance and overall posture.

These interoceptive senses are the ones that are referred to in the term 'faulty sensory appreciation', but why, when and how did they become faulty? The answer is perhaps two-fold: firstly, we now have so many more stimuli directed towards the five outward senses that the information from the inner senses is suppressed or screened out by the overwhelmed brain. Secondly, if our muscles are constantly in a state of tension, it seems that these internal senses cannot work efficiently. As a result, the interoceptive senses become unreliable and begin to give us faulty information about where we are in space. As this tension becomes more and more ingrained, we can become totally unaware of how or what we are doing. Eventually, many of us are continuously reacting to false information as to where we are in space and what we are doing at any given time. In other words, we get caught in a vicious cycle: we cannot feel our own muscle tension because our feedback senses are not working properly, and our feedback senses are not working properly because of our muscle tension. The first thing we need to do is to find out exactly which muscles are over-tensing as we go about our daily activities. We can do this by bringing our awareness to everyday actions and beginning to consciously release the muscle tension that is at the heart of the problem. Usually we don't give a moment's thought as to how we move; we simply move in the way that feels *normal, comfortable* and *right* to us. Yet this is the main problem: our habits of reacting to stimuli will invariably feel totally normal, comfortable and right to us, yet they are often the root cause of our poor posture or health problem.

Without realizing it, many of us take our poor postural habits and faulty sensory appreciation into every action we perform, with catastrophic consequences. Even worse, we often bring those habits and faulty sensory appreciation into our practice of various forms of physical exercise, such as yoga, Pilates, physiotherapy exercises, martial arts, gym work, running and various sports. If an activity that is supposed to be good for us is done with far too much tension, we can cause ourselves injury, ironically while we are trying to keep fit.

Over the last 25 years I have talked to a great many doctors, physiotherapists, fitness and sports instructors, yoga and Pilates teachers, manual-handling trainers and ergonomic instructors, yet very few of them were even aware of the existence of faulty sensory appreciation. This is very serious indeed, because with all good faith we may be carrying out a series of instructions, but performing them totally incorrectly and could well be

      “ The Alexander Technique will benefit anyone
        whether they are an elite athlete or whether they just
        wish to live life without the aches and pains that
        many people suffer and accept as part of life. It is a
        pity that these techniques are not shown to us all at
        an early age for I have no doubt that this would
        alleviate many of the causes of ill health in our
        communities. ”

Greg Chappell, Australian test cricketer (1970–84)

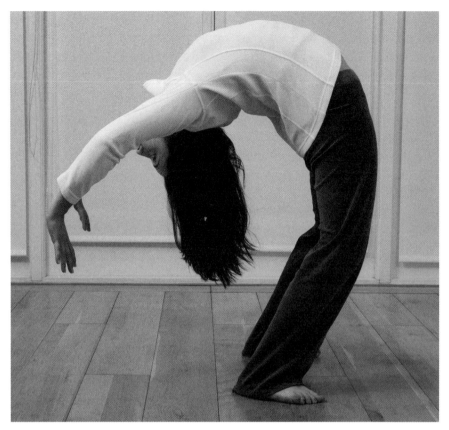

32: Due to inactive lifestyles, such as sitting for long periods at an office desk, many people resort to 'goal-oriented' exercises, which overstrain the body, causing even more tension. The increase in the numbers of sports injury clinics opening (where people go after they damage themselves while trying to get fit!) testifies to this fact.

causing ourselves harm. A good example of this is in the manual-handling instruction when lifting. Many people are taught that the way to lift is to 'bend the knees and keep the back straight', and it's easy to misinterpret this instruction to mean 'keep the back vertical' or 'keep the back rigid'. So, many nurses and care-workers try to lift heavy patients while trying to keep their backs vertical, and as a result can develop serious back problems. Just look at young children: every time they bend to pick something up, they always bend their knees, hips and ankle joints and although their back stays beautifully straight, it is not vertical – in fact, quite often it is 45 degrees forward from vertical.

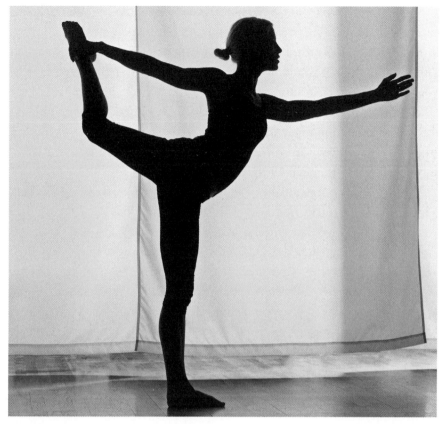

33: When doing any form of exercise, make sure that you are in balance and you are conscious of the way you use yourself while you are performing the activity. When having Alexander lessons, ask your teacher to examine the way that you perform your exercise regime.

The only reliable way of finding out what we are actually doing is to seek verification by external means, such as by using mirrors, a video-recorder or guidance from an Alexander teacher. It is only by getting reliable feedback that we can have a chance to first see and then relinquish our harmful habits. For all we know we may be leaning backwards, forwards or sideways when we stand or sit, but be absolutely convinced that we are perfectly straight. A good example can be found at any hair salon: when a hairdresser tells a client to put their head straight, they often put their head to one side and the hairdresser then has to manually straighten the head for them, after which many people feel as though their head is lopsided.

You can try the following observation exercises at home in order to gain a practical understanding of faulty sensory appreciation:

Stand side-on to a mirror and *without looking in the mirror* stand in what you think is an upright position. Make sure that you are standing as straight as you possibly can. Then turn your head only and check in the mirror to see whether your feelings of being straight match the reality. If they do not, use the mirror to stand in a way that is straight. Now ask yourself: Does this feel straight? Use a second mirror if you have one so that you do not have to move your body too much when observing.

Now try looking straight ahead and, *without looking at your feet*, place them about 30cm (12in) apart from the inside. Still without looking at them, place your feet parallel to each other, if they are not already this way. Both feet should be pointing straight ahead. Now look at your feet to check if their actual position matches your inner sense of their position. If not, you are experiencing what Alexander meant by 'faulty sensory appreciation'.

Next you can look at your feet as you place them parallel with one another and 30 cm (12 in) apart. Close your eyes and notice how they feel. Do they feel parallel? If not, again you are experiencing faulty sensory appreciation.

Body mapping

A somewhat related subject to faulty sensory appreciation is that of 'body mapping', which explores our mental image of our own bodies. Our 'body map' is influenced by the way we think we are constructed rather than how we are actually designed. Body mapping was first described by William Conable, Alexander teacher and professor of cello at the Ohio State University School of Music. He derived the whole concept of body mapping by observing the way his music students moved while playing their instruments. He noticed that students would nearly always move according to how they thought they were structured rather than according to reality. When he was able to show his students how they were actually anatomically designed, their movement in playing became efficient, expressive and appropriate for the task required. His wife, Barbara, then developed the body-mapping work by writing books and training others.

While teaching the Alexander Technique to musicians, both William and Barbara realized that there was a great deal of confusion among their students about how the body worked and the actual position and size of certain bones, joints and muscles. They realized that by having a clearer idea about the way the body's mechanisms function anatomically, people can learn to let go of certain postural habits more quickly. If we have an incorrect map of ourselves, we can easily be thrown off balance. If we can start to think of having good balance as synonymous with having good posture, then by improving one, we will often help the other. It might be useful for you to have some anatomical drawings or illustrations available as you read through the information below. These can be obtained from a library or the internet.

Head–spine or neck joint

It is important to know what Alexander meant when he referred to the neck; he was talking about the area where the atlanto-occipital and the atlas-axis joints are located.

The atlanto-occipital joint

This Articulates between the top of the spine (atlas) and the base of the skull (occipital bone), and allows the forward and backward (nodding) movement of the head.

The head–spine joint is one of the main joints in the body, and the freedom of this joint is crucial to the proper functioning of the Primary Control. When asked to locate the position of this joint, many people think that it is at the back of the head, or even at the top of their shoulders. In reality, the atlanto-occipital joint is located between the ear holes, and it is very important to think of the top of the neck being between the ears when directing the neck to be free. It will be much harder or even impossible to obtain a free neck if you are wrongly mapping this joint (*See* photo 34).

Arm–body joint

Most people imagine that the bones of their arm connect to their body at the outside point of their shoulder. This is because when we look in the mirror it appears that this is exactly where the arms meet the body, but this is actually incorrect. In reality, the bones of the arm continue under the skin and muscle and actually connect onto the sternum. The upper arm (*humerus*) is connected only to the shoulder blade (*scapula*), which in turn is connected to

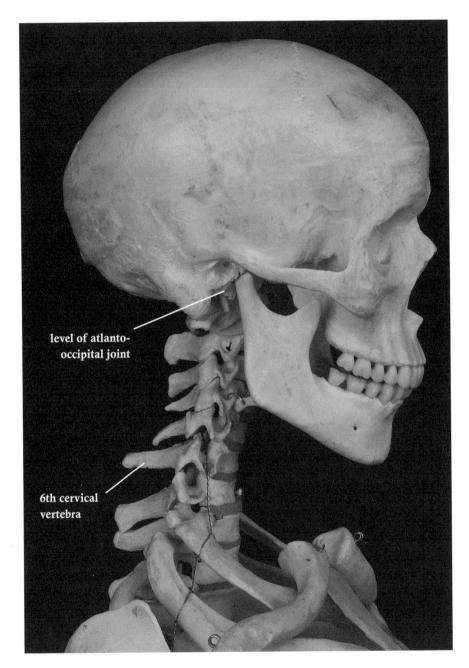

level of atlanto-occipital joint

6th cervical vertebra

34: Many people map the joint between the head and spine (the atlanto-occipital joint) as being just above the shoulders, whereas it is approximately level with the ear holes.

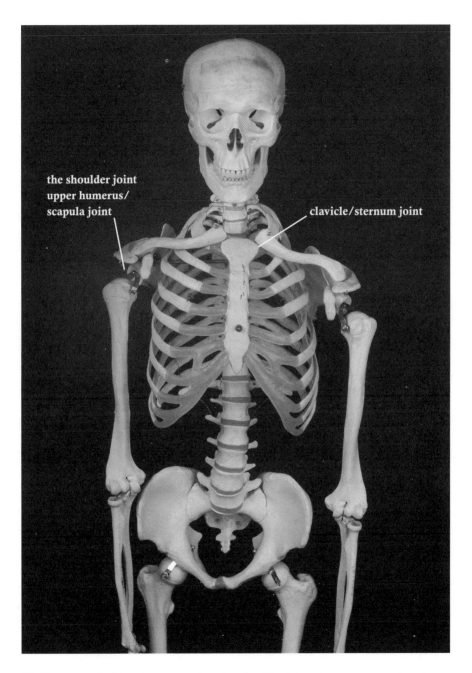

the shoulder joint
upper humerus/
scapula joint

clavicle/sternum joint

35: Many people think the arm ends at the shoulder joint. As you can see from the photo here, the bones of the arm include the shoulder blade (scapula) and collarbone (clavicle) as well. So, in fact, the arm ends at the sternum – quite a distance from the shoulder joint.

the collarbone (*clavicle*). It is where the collarbone meets the breastbone (*sternum*) that the arm actually joins the rest of the body (*see* photo 35). The arms are therefore, in effect, only 2.5–5cm (1–2in) away from each other. We therefore have five joints of the arm (wrist joint, elbow joint, upper arm to shoulder blade joint, shoulder blade to collarbone joint, and collarbone to breastbone joint), and not three joints as is commonly believed. You can test this out by placing the fingers of your right hand on the left collarbone and then raising your left arm so that your fingers are pointing up to the sky; you should clearly feel the collarbone moving.

Hip joint

Mis-mapping of the body often continues when it comes to finding the location of the hip joint. If you ask most people where their hip joint is, they will point to the top of the pelvis, usually in the region of the bone that protrudes at the side (*iliac crest*). This is not, however, where the joint is at all, but it is often where people bend from. The actual joint is situated lower and further into the body and is, in fact, situated in the groin area. When people bend down, however, they will usually try to bend from where they *think* the hip joint is (at the top of the iliac crest). Consequently, they will try to bend the spine (around the area of the lumbar 4th and 5th vertebrae) rather than the hip joint. This action can lead to many lower back problems, especially around the area of Lumbar 4 and Lumbar 5 and the sacro-iliac joints, which all come under pressure when bending in the wrong place.

The spine

If you ask people to draw the shape of the spine, many will draw the spine in a gentle S shape. While this is accurate when standing, the spine actually changes shape depending on what you are doing. When you're sitting or bending your knees, the lumbar area loses some of its curve and becomes much straighter. Observing a domestic cat is useful to understand this point. Its spine will take on different shapes in different situations. When eating its food, the cat's spine is very straight, and when it is lying in front of the fire its spine is very rounded. When stretching, the cat will arch its back. In the same way, our spine changes shape, depending on what we are doing. Observe how the shape of the spine of children playing on a beach changes. I have found that the lumbar supports found in cars and back shops can encourage

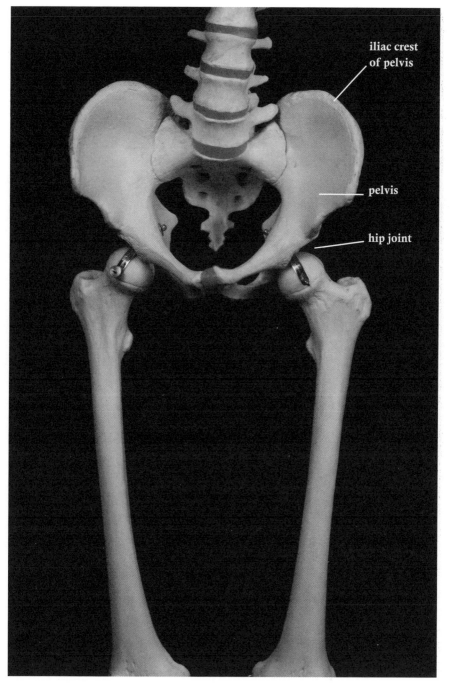

iliac crest
of pelvis

pelvis

hip joint

36: Many people mistakenly think that the ball and socket joint between the leg and pelvis is at the top of the pelvis, whereas it is, in fact, much lower.

an over-arching of the lumbar spine and can actually exacerbate lower back problems rather than bringing relief.

The spine is mainly designed for turning or rotary movements, rather than a bending movement, yet many people tend to overarch their lumbar curve, causing a major restriction in any rotational movements. Again, just observe young children or pre-industrialized people and you will see that they typically keep their spines totally straight even when reaching for something on the ground, yet they freely rotate their spines. Over-bending the spine forwards or backwards is often a gross misuse of the body and can put huge pressure on the intervertebral discs. If this way of bending becomes a habit, it can cause major health problems.

The length of the spine is also often misunderstood: it is a very long structure extending from the ears to beneath the hip joint.

Awareness

So the key to improving your posture in everyday actions is to become more conscious of what you are actually doing and thinking. Many of us have had incorrect training when it comes to posture, and that training needs to be undone. In the next chapter we will have a look at basic everyday activities like sitting and standing to see if we can improve them.

CHAPTER 10

Your Inner Acrobat

The most important human endeavour is the striving for morality in our actions. Our inner balance and even our very existence depend on it. Only morality in our actions can give beauty and dignity to life.

Albert Einstein

During his lifetime, Alexander admired the way that acrobatic performers used themselves while both keeping still and moving. He noticed that these performers, whether on or off the stage, moved with the maximum efficiency and gracefulness.

Acrobats have learnt to be in harmony with gravity, as they need to be perfectly balanced in all the actions that they perform, and as a consequence have an elegance and poise similar to that of young children. Acrobats use gravity to help them in many of their awe-inspiring acts. This is also true for the surfer, skater and dancer, because balance and fine coordination are of the essence. While the acrobat lives life in balance and working with gravity, many of us, in contrast, are constantly fighting gravity with excessive muscle tension in our every waking moment. This tension becomes so habitually ingrained over the years that we even tense our muscles while asleep, evidenced by the common problem of grinding teeth at night. In fact, poor posture has become so common that it is now perceived as normal, so much so that it has become striking when we see a person with an upright and balanced posture.

Since the mind, emotions and body are, in essence, all the same thing, when we are in balance so too are our emotions (which we experience as

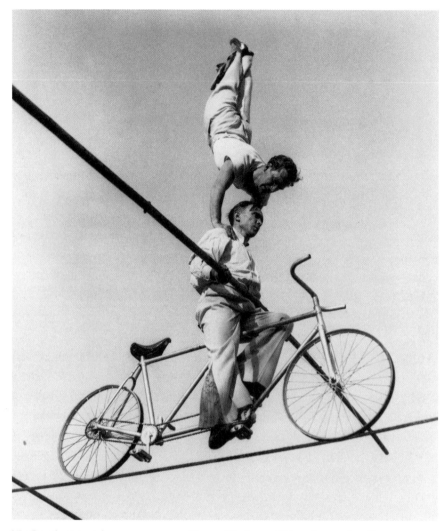

37: Good posture is synonymous with good balance. When improving the way you use yourself, it can be helpful to be aware of how your head is balanced on top of your spine.

calmness) and our minds (which we experience as metal composure). So moving in balance can produce calmness on other levels too. Our posture is really the sum of thousands of thoughts we make each and every day, and by changing these thoughts, while walking, sitting and bending, we can see and feel a profound effect on our overall wellbeing. The American Trappist monk Thomas Merton once said: 'Happiness is not a matter of intensity, but of balance, order, rhythm and harmony.' By bringing balance, order, rhythm and harmony into our everyday movements, we will not only be improving our posture but we will be bringing our whole life back into balance.

The Secret to Good Balance: the Primary Control

The human body is, in fact, an amazing anti-gravity mechanism, which is delicately balanced by a series of intricate reflexes and internal feedback mechanisms that continuously inform the brain. This, in turn, organizes our movement in perfect balance, without any conscious effort on our part. If we begin to lose balance, the right mechanisms immediately come into play to restore our equilibrium. The habit of over-tensing muscles severely interferes with this natural organization.

Let us consider the human body for a moment: it is one of, if not the most, unstable structures living on the planet. We consist of over 650 muscles and 206 bones, all of irregular shapes, constantly balanced one on top of another. Right at the bottom we have arched feet, which support the lower legs, which in turn support the upper legs, and on top of the legs balances the pelvis. These structures are made up of joints and incredible mechanisms comprising a rounded bone balancing on another rounded bone, (which can be clearly seen in the case of the ankle, knee and hip joints. Further up the body we have the spine, balancing on the pelvis, which itself comprises 24 vertebrae, which are placed one on top of the other. And if that is not the most amazing balancing act you have ever seen, right on top of the spine sits the head, which is finely balanced and on average weighs about 4.5 kg (10 lb). It does not take much to see that not only is the human body inherently unstable, but also that we are very, very top-heavy, and therefore we require little or no effort to move, but conversely we require a lot of effort to maintain a position or fixed posture. So in reality we are all acrobats, and even standing consists of several balancing acts at any given time; this is, in fact, one of nature's most amazing miracles. So if we are ever to have good posture we need to develop a good sense of balance! Einstein once said 'To keep your balance you must keep moving' and good posture is all about movement and not about position.

Not only does the weight of the head cause us to be 'top-heavy', it is actually set off-balance on top of our spines. It is set in such a way that if we

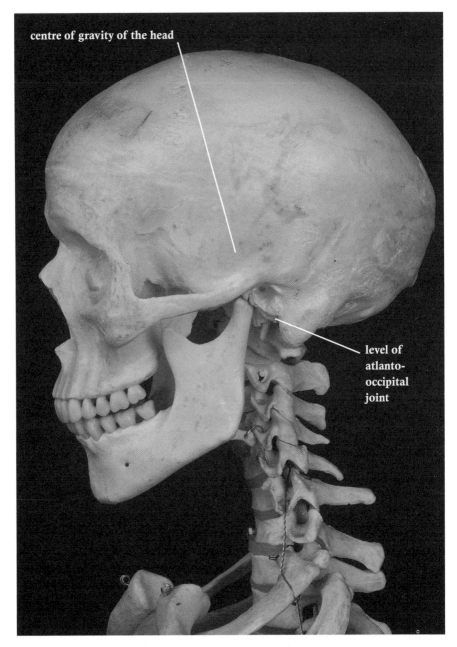

centre of gravity of the head

level of
atlanto-
occipital
joint

38: The centre of gravity of the head is situated forward of the balancing point
(atlanto-occipital joint). This means that we are designed to move by releasing
tension rather than increasing tension. By learning the Alexander Technique many
people say they feel their movements are lighter as they realize that they hardly need
any effort to perform everyday tasks.

relax the neck muscles, the head is inclined to drop forwards. If you watch someone falling asleep while sitting in a chair, you'll notice that the head invariably drops forward and down onto the chest. So not only are we trying to balance the relatively heavy weight of the head on the spine, but we are also coping with the fact that its point of balance is not under its centre of gravity (*See* photo 38).

At first this might sound confusing, until you realize that the reason that the pivot point of the head is behind its centre of gravity is to make movement effortless. All we have to do to move is to release the muscles surrounding the neck joint (the atlanto-occipital joint) by allowing the neck to be free. The head will then go slightly forward on the spine in an upward direction, and this slight forward adjustment of the head will take the rest of the body into movement, as long as there is freedom in all the other 'hinge' joints (ankles, knees and hip joints). In other words, in order to move, a human being has only to let go of the tension in certain muscles and a complex reflex system will do the rest. Most other movements require effort, and the maximum effort is needed at the beginning of the action. For example, a car or aeroplane needs most power when it accelerates from a stationary position; it needs much less energy to keep it going at a constant speed. The human body, on the other hand, needs no effort to move and actually requires a release of muscle tension. Once the head begins to move forwards, the body will naturally follow, and the reflexes then spring into operation as a response to the movement. In short, the relative position of the head in relation to the neck and back controls, organizes and guides all our movements for us with little or no effort on our part. When the head is not balanced, the Primary Control, as Alexander called it, ceases to work effectively or efficiently. You will need an Alexander teacher to show you this as it is difficult to experience this on your own.

❝ I love the Alexander Technique. It has corrected my posture, improved my health and changed my life. ❞

Alec McCowen CBE, actor

Eyes

To maintain this balance it is important to be aware of how you use your eyes. It is a common habit for people to look down by letting the whole head and neck drop, rather than looking down just with the eyes and keeping the head lightly balanced on top. You become aware right now as you are reading this book: are you looking down with your eyes or the whole head? In my own teaching I have also found that many people can dramatically

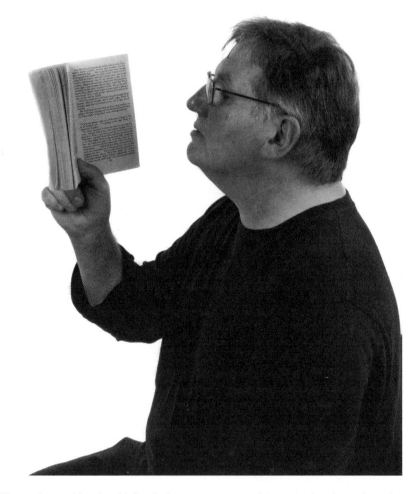

39: When using varifocal or bi-focal glasses, many people unconsciously get into the habit of pulling their head back onto their spine when reading. This can often become a habit and consequently lead to neck problems and tension headaches.

alter the balance of the head when wearing varifocal or bi-focal glasses, and tend to pull their head back when reading so that they can look through the part of the lens that is suitable; without knowing it, they are probably giving themselves chronic neck problems. If you are one of these people, the Technique can help you to become aware of the habit and learn to read in different way.

Standing

It is important to recognize that standing is an activity rather than a position. If you watch a young child standing, you will see that they are not actually still, but swaying very gently in balance. They are not doing so consciously: their reflexes are. Adults, on the other hand, often stand in fixed positions, but the effect of deliberately 'standing up straight' and 'pulling our shoulders back' is to pull us off balance and is therefore detrimental to good posture. As we saw in the last chapter, standing in a straight position might also not be as easy as we think, as we cannot feel with our internal senses what is straight and what is not. The only real way to tell when we are balanced and when we are not is by means of the weight distribution in the feet. If we are unbalanced, the weight will be thrown onto the front, back, insides or outsides of our feet, and just by noticing where this distribution of weight is, we can become much more aware of how we are standing, even when we do not have a mirror to directly inform us of the reality. When standing, the weight distribution should be on three points of each foot, and this brings a certain amount of balance. The first point is the heel, the second is the ball of the foot and the third is situated on the outside of the foot at the beginning of the little toe. If you are habitually standing on only two or even one of these three points, you will be less balanced, and consequently you will need to tense many more muscles to keep you upright.

Remove your shoes and stand up as you usually do while you are reading these words. Ask yourself whether you are standing more on one foot than the other, or are you equally balanced on both of your feet? Even if you find you are equally balanced on both your feet, ask yourself if this is your usual way of standing, and, if not, stand in a way that feels normal to you and then ask yourself the same questions again.

Now see if you are standing more on your heels or more on the balls of your feet, as this will help to indicate whether you are leaning backwards or forwards. Similarly, see if you are standing more on the outside or on the inside of your feet, and remember that this can be different for each foot. The habit of standing more on the inside of your feet can produce 'flat feet', which is the outward sign of the habit of pulling your body down and the knees towards each other. Lastly, ask yourself if your knees are locked back with excessive tension, or if they are over-relaxed so that your knees are bent?

By asking these questions, you can begin to notice your own habitual way of standing and decide whether it is balanced or unbalanced. We can improve our standing by being conscious of the way we stand and by making sure our feet are making even contact with the ground. It can also be a good idea to observe the way other people stand in shops and banks when waiting in a queue, as this can increase your general awareness.

Improved standing

There is no one right or correct way of standing, and, in fact, there are many ways of standing that do not put undue pressure on the body. An important characteristic of a beneficial way of standing is that it is balanced. Alexander did not advocate any one correct way of standing, as he maintained that this would only encourage a new set of habits, but he did give his pupils useful suggestions to remember while standing:

1. Place the feet approximately 30cm (12in) apart, as this immediately gives a more stable base on which to support the rest of the body. *Note*: this measurement is from the inside of the feet; so for tall people the feet need to be a little further apart and for short people a little closer together.

2. When standing for long periods, it is helpful to take one foot approximately 15cm (6in) back, so that about 60 per cent of the weight of the body is resting on the rear foot. Place the feet with an angle of approximately 45 degrees between them. This helps to prevent the all-too-common habit of sinking down into one hip, which can affect the balance and coordination of the whole structure of your body.

40: The unbalanced way in which we stand may also cause excessive tension throughout the body, leading to a variety of back, neck, hip, knee and foot problems.

41: By placing your feet a little way apart, with one slightly behind the other, as shown, you can stand in a much more balanced way. This in turn can dramatically reduce tension and can alleviate an array of muscular or skeletal problems.

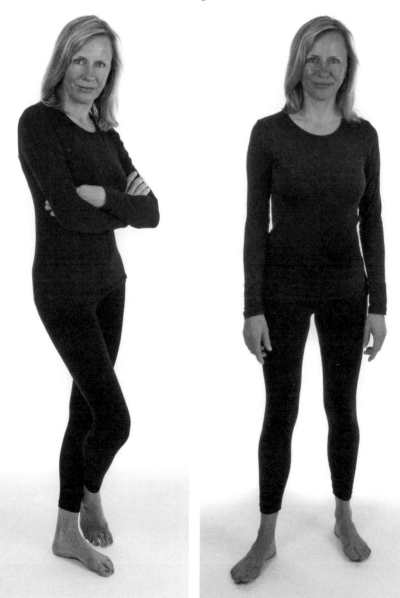

3. If you notice that you are pushing your pelvis forward, imagine it gently releasing back without deliberately throwing the body too far forward (make sure you are allowing your neck to be free and your head to move forward and up and your spine to lengthen at the same time). This helps to eliminate the very common tendency of over-arching the back when in a standing position. *Note*: make sure you are only thinking and not actually doing this action.

Sitting

Compared to our grandparents, we spend many more hours a day sitting in chairs. It is a good idea to separate sitting into two distinct categories: sitting for relaxation and sitting in activity. While you are sitting for relaxation, for example, when using a reclining chair or a sofa or armchair while watching TV, you only need to let the chair fully support you, so that no one part of your body has to bear undue pressure or tension. You can always use cushions to support your head if you need to.

Sitting while in activity is a different matter altogether, and sitting at a desk or table while working or eating requires us to be balanced on the two sitting bones and feet. Make sure that you have even support on all these four areas, and when you are leaning forward at a desk or table, do not bend your spine, but rather use your hip joints and sitting bones to help you to transfer weight from the sitting bones onto the feet. When moving back away from the desk, just reverse the process and transfer your weight back over your sitting bones. While you are sitting during any activity, try to be balanced, poised and movable rather than hold any one fixed position. Last but not least, make sure your chair is well designed. (*See also* chapter 8 on posture and furniture.)

Bending down

Bending down is yet another amazing balancing act! When bending down to pick objects up, many people do not bend their knees sufficiently – and sometimes not at all. Often you will see people actually bending at the waist, where in fact there is no hinge joint, so in reality they are bending their spine.

42: The full effects of the misuse of ourselves can easily be seen in this X-ray image of a person working at a computer. This person, like many others, is completely unaware of the damage he is doing to himself.

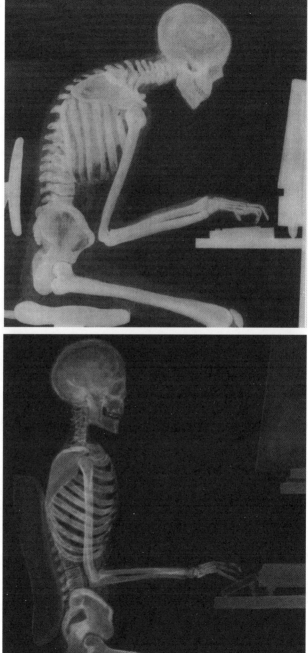

43: By learning the Alexander Technique, we can regain our natural poise and balance while performing simple everyday tasks such as working at our desks, and so avoid a multitude of health problems in later life.

44: Many people in developed countries bend their backs instead of the knee, hip and ankle joints when picking up objects. This is not how nature designed us to work and this way of moving can lead to a wide range of muscular or skeletal problems, such as back pain, later in life.

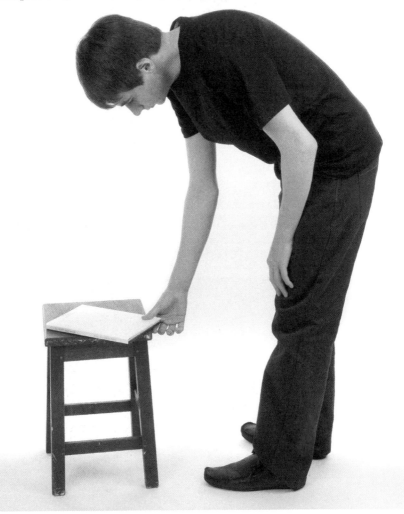

This can cause not only direct damage to the spine, but also the body to be completely out of balance, immediately putting enormous strain on the entire muscular system, especially the back, thigh and neck muscles, which have to tighten to prevent the person falling over. The crucial point here is that, without realizing it, they are actually lifting more than half their body weight every time they straighten up from bending to pick up even a light

45: By the use of inhibition and direction, we can learn to choose a different way of moving, which puts less strain on ourselves.

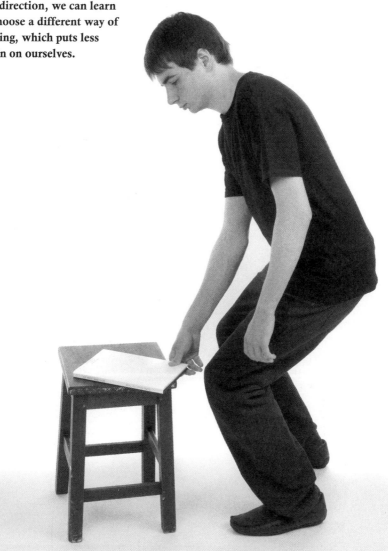

object, which causes even further muscular tension. This sort of misuse is a disaster for the body, and, if habitual, can often directly cause lower back pain and neck problems. Furthermore, all the internal organs are put under pressure and breathing is restricted. If you ever watch young children, indigenous people or professional weightlifters, you will see that they squat when bending, using their very powerful leg muscles. You will rarely see young children or indigenous people bending down without bending their hips, knees and ankles. Some time ago I heard an interesting story about some missionaries who went to Africa and mixed with some native people. The native people were awestruck by the fact that the white missionaries often bent down from the waist without bending their knees, and so they gave them an African name, which, when directly translated, meant 'the tribe without knees'! All joints require natural and regular movement to keep them healthy, so by using your major joints in order to maintain balance and equilibrium, you will also be keeping your joints free from problems and your muscles perfectly toned.

Try picking a magazine off a coffee table in your usual way and stop just as your hand reaches it. Ask yourself the following questions: Are your knees bending? If so, by how much? Do you feel in balance or unbalanced? Can you feel any tension in your body, and, if so, where? How much overall effort are you using in this simple activity?

Now repeat the same action, only this time make a conscious decision to make sure you allow freedom in your neck so that your head can move forward and up and your spine can lengthen. At the same time, allow your knees to bend so that they go forward and away from each other. Allow them to bend more than you normally would, but make sure that you are not pulling them in towards one another. Does this feel more balanced and easier on your muscles and joints? You will help yourself to improve overall posture overnight if you start to use the hip, knee and ankle joints as nature intended in order to keep you balanced in the hundreds of actions you perform every day. Remember, new ways of moving will feel strange at first.

Moving from sitting to standing

Many of us make a big deal about getting out of a chair. This is because we have an idea that we are trying to leave the chair in a vertical fashion, and by doing this we think of ourselves as having to fight gravity, putting enormous strain on our entire structure. But getting out of a chair is simply transferring your weight from the chair onto the feet and can feel effortless if we use the body's natural mechanisms and reflexes. After you have had a few Alexander lessons, you might like to try this following procedure: first, try getting up slowly in your usual way and see if you can feel the stresses and strains in your legs, neck, back or feet. Now do it again slowly, following these simple instructions:

1. Make sure that your feet are a little apart and not too far forward. Your knee should be roughly above the front of your foot.

2. As you begin to stand up, allow your head to move first by allowing it to go slightly forward and up away from your shoulders, then allow the rest of your body to follow.

3. While moving, think of the back lengthening. Make sure your neck does not drop downwards or your head get pulled back (thinking of your head moving away from your pelvis will help).

4. Only bend forward in the area of the sitting bones or the hip joint by 'hinging' at the hip joint and not at waist level. (*See* photo 36, page 113).

5. As more weight goes onto your feet, you will feel an increased pressure under the feet, which triggers your postural reflexes, and you will begin to leave the chair spontaneously and with little effort.

6. As you leave the chair, allow most of your weight to go through the heels, thinking of your hips, knees and ankles 'unbending', rather than straighten the legs by over-tensing your leg muscles and pushing your feet into the floor.

If this is done in a balanced way, you should be able to pause at any moment with grace and ease and feel totally balanced.

Moving from standing to sitting

A common habit that many of us have is to fall backwards when sitting down. This immediately unduly excites what Alexander called our fear reflexes and causes the head to retract backwards, the shoulders to hunch and the back to over-arch, because the body senses it is off balance and tries to protect itself. Again, if this is the habitual way we sit down, the body will retain this tension unconsciously, and the neck, shoulders and back can remain permanently in a state of tension. The natural way to sit down is to allow the head to move forward (without allowing the neck to drop down) and at the same time to bend the hips, knees and ankle joints so that you descend in perfect balance. Again, you should be able to pause at any moment and balance with ease. As your sitting bones reach the chair, allow them to roll back, keeping your head balanced and your back in a lengthened state. If you are really in balance, you will be able to change your mind and get up at any time you want to without making any effort. It is essential to realize that the instruction of the 'head going forward' is in relation to the top of the spine and *not* in space. It is not 'face forward' but the whole of the head; thinking of your nose dropping minutely can be helpful.

So by thinking about the balance of your body as a whole during your activities, you will be accessing your inner acrobat. This will naturally improve your sense of physical integrity, improving your posture, poise and grace of movement. And don't forget that you are doing a balancing act of your head resting on top of your spine wherever you go!

CHAPTER 11

Inside Yourself

The real voyage of discovery consists not in seeking new landscapes, but in having new eyes.

Marcel Proust

There are many ways that you can begin to help yourself at home. As you saw earlier, Alexander used mirrors to help him solve his problem, and you can do the same. The Alexander Technique consists of inhibition and direction, and it would be very helpful to keep this in mind as you are following the next few awareness exercises. It is vital that you do not try to directly bring about the change in your posture by tensing your muscles even further, which is what many people do. Observation, without immediately *doing* anything, is an important key to learning the Technique.

Awareness exercise 1: Initial observation

Choose a quiet time of day when you can be alone. It does not matter whether it is early in the morning, during the day or in the evening. Spend a few minutes lying down and gently bring your awareness to your body. You might like to start with your feet and work upwards. *Without trying to 'do' anything*, see if you can be aware of any tension in the foot, toes or ankle. After a minute or so, begin to bring your awareness to the legs and then progressively upwards to your pelvis, back, arms, neck and finally your head. Take as much time as you feel you need with any particular part of your body. Practise being an impartial observer of yourself, but make no negative judgement on what you are feeling or thinking.

This exploration procedure can also be done sitting or standing, and different positions can bring about different observations. As outlined earlier, it is important that you just observe to begin with without wanting to change anything. Some people, however, find that by just observing, a certain amount of their tension releases spontaneously. By observing in this way, you can start to build a picture of where you hold most of your tension. It's useful to keep notes of your experiences and observations.

Many of us think of posture as only external, but it actually can affect the inside of the body just as much. Our internal organs can be squeezed by the over-tightening of the muscular system; we can squash our lungs until we are barely getting enough air; we can tense our muscles so much that we trap our own nerves; we can clench the jaw so hard that we wear down our teeth; and we can pull bone down on bone, causing a variety of 'wear and tear' conditions in later life. Amazingly, all this is done without our knowing.

The muscular system accounts, on average, for 40 per cent of our body weight and consists of more than 650 muscles. We have muscles on the *inside* of the ribcage (the transversus thoracis, which is underneath the sternum and front ribs) and even in the inner ear (the tensor tympani and the stapedius muscle). The tongue is a muscle, as is the heart. In fact, the muscular system can be found almost everywhere in the body.

Awareness exercise 2: Observing the inside of yourself

Again, choose a quiet time and place.
Become aware of your tongue – is it doing anything or is it quietly resting on the floor of your mouth?
Are you clenching the jaw muscles or are they at peace?
Can you become aware of the muscles around your ribcage, and are they tight or free? Are they causing any restriction in your breathing? Are your ribs moving or fixed?
Can you feel any muscular tension in your body causing you to pull inwards or contract your structure?

Take a journey inside your whole body and see if you can start to be aware of how your muscles are working. Perhaps they are working too hard, or perhaps they are not working hard enough. Becoming aware of how our muscles pull us out of shape can be very beneficial to the process of improving posture and the way we move.

Awareness exercise 3: Mirror observation

The aim of this exercise is for you to see your own tension. You can perform the exercise first sitting and then standing. You will be using your sense of *proprioception* (the internal sense that gives you feedback as to the position of the parts of your body in relationship to one another). Even if you are blindfolded, you are aware through proprioception whether your arm is above your head or hanging by your side. Proprioception gives you vital information as to whether you are straight or leaning backwards, forwards or sideways. Place a mirror in front of you, close your eyes and try to 'feel' what shape you are standing or sitting in. After a minute or so, open your eyes and see if your actual position is the same as what you imagined. Also notice if one shoulder is higher than the other, or if they are both raised, or if your legs or feet are pulling inwards. Also try moving the mirror to the side of you, as you can see more clearly if you are leaning backwards or forwards. Again, make a note of your observations, as these can change day by day. If you repeat this exercise over several days, you will probably be able to notice more and more patterns or tendencies.

Directions

As we saw earlier in the book, Alexander came up with the idea of giving himself mental orders, which he called 'directions', to help change his unconscious harmful postural habits. He first created a space, which he called 'inhibition', between stimulus and response. He did this in order to prevent his unconscious habitual patterns from repeating themselves in an 'automatic' way. He then began to give conscious mental instructions (directions) to the part of the body that he had been unable to control before. In his book *The Use of the Self* he described 'giving directions' as: 'A process which involves projecting messages from the brain to the body's mechanisms and conducting the energy necessary for the use of these mechanisms.'

Merely thinking creates activity in the brain without adding to physical tension. We can actually change our posture and the entire way we use ourselves with our thoughts. One of the reasons this is possible is that from a neuroscientific point of view, imagining an action and actually performing it are not very different. When people close their eyes and visualize an object, the primary visual cortex lights up in the same way as if the person was seeing that object in real life. In a study published in the *Journal of Neuropsychology*, Dr Guang Yue and Dr Kelly Cole had one group of participants exercise a finger for a month, while another group just imagined exercising the same finger. The result showed that the group that performed the physical exercise gained strength in the finger by 30 per cent, while the group who were just imagining the exercise gained finger strength of 22 per cent. This scientifically demonstrates the power of thinking can change the physical body. So when giving mental orders or directions, you are directly influencing the entire way you use yourself, including your posture, whether you 'feel' anything happening or not. You can prove this to yourself by signing your name and then visualizing signing it – it takes roughly the same time. Now try visualizing signing your name with the other hand and you will usually find that it takes much longer; about the time it would take in

“ The Alexander Technique can be sustaining; it is something that if learned well, can be carried along with you for the rest of your life. It gives you confidence to be who you are when you are up in front of an audience. ”

Patrick Maddams, Managing Director, Royal Academy of Music

real life. The more you think or visualize the directions, the better you get at doing it, and the time it takes becomes shorter and shorter.

In the next procedure we are going to look at how to start projecting these directions, or orders, to bring about a release of tension. It is possible to direct *specific* parts of yourself (for example, you can think of your fingers lengthening) or you can direct your *whole* self (such as when thinking of your entire structure lengthening). It is important to remember that these 'directions' are only thoughts. It is very common for people to try and 'do' the directions rather than just think them, and without realizing it, they can be adding to the tension, which only makes matters worse. Alexander was known to have said that there is no such thing as right position, but there is such a thing as right direction, and it is worth remembering that when you are trying to improve your posture. Directions tend to be expansive, spacious, wide, free, roomy and open; they are the perfect antidote to poor posture, which tends to be narrow, contracted, restricted, constricted, confined, pulled down and pulled in. During Alexander lessons, the teacher will show you how to give yourself directions.

The Primary Control

The primary cause of poor posture is over-tightening of the neck muscles, which interferes with what Alexander called the 'Primary Control'. This can throw the whole body out of balance. Alexander realized that the priority was to achieve a reduction of tension in the neck area by allowing the neck to be free, so that the Primary Control could work more efficiently. So the primary direction is:

- Allow the neck to be free *in such a way that*

- the head can go forward and upward *in order that*

- the back can lengthen and widen.

Allow the neck to be free

The main purpose of this instruction is to eliminate the excess tension that is almost always present in the muscles of the neck. If we are ever going to have good posture, it is essential that the head must be allowed to move freely on the spine. This should always be the first part of the direction given, because unless the Primary Control is able to organize the rest of the body without hindrance, the rest of the direction will be relatively ineffective. As we saw in Chapter 9, the joint where the head meets the spine is directly between the ear holes.

Allow the head to go forward and upward

This tells you *in which way* the neck needs to be free. If you just thought of your neck being free without an upward direction, the head would probably fall downwards. The movement forwards is often so small that it is hardly detectable and really only prevents the head from pulling backwards. This part of the direction helps to keep the head finely balanced, ready to take the rest of the body into movement, which allows all the mechanisms of the body to function naturally and freely. It is important to realize that the forward direction is the head going forward *on the spine* (as if you are about to nod your head affirmatively) and not forward in space (like putting your *face* forwards to peer at the TV). The upward direction of the head is always *the crown of your head away from the spine* and not away from the ground, although these will be the same when you are upright.

Allow the back to lengthen and widen

When the spine lengthens, it helps to straighten and align itself and can reduce any over-curvature that may have occurred through misuse. Sometimes this lengthening can cause a narrowing of the back to occur, and thinking of the back widening helps to prevent this.

This primary direction is actually very simple and straightforward. However, because of our unreliable kinaesthesia, it can be confusing when first practised. It is good to remember that because we live in a fast-moving world, when results do not happen immediately we presume that we are doing something wrong or that the Technique is not working. Be patient and observant, and realize that changing the habits of a lifetime does take time. It is strongly advised that when you start giving directions you have at least a few lessons from a registered Alexander teacher to make sure you are on the right track.

Secondary directions

The primary direction, as described earlier in this chapter, is 'Allow the neck to be free, in such a way that the head can go forward and upward, in order that the back can lengthen and widen'. Whereas this can be applied universally, secondary directions may be applied to certain conditions or ailments. For example, if a person comes to me suffering from rounded shoulders, I may give them an instruction to: 'Think of your shoulders going away from each other'; or if someone comes to me with arthritic fingers, I may ask them to: 'Think of your fingers lengthening'. Some people just think or repeat the words to themselves, while others actually have a three- dimensional image in their head. Use whatever method is best for you. Here are some directions that you may find useful:

- Think of your fingers lengthening and the palms of your hands widening.

- Think of your shoulders releasing away from one another.

- Think of your left shoulder releasing away from your right hip.

- Think of your right shoulder releasing away from your left hip.

- Think of your elbows releasing away from one another.

- Think of your toes lengthening as the soles of your feet spread out on to the floor. (This is a common area of tension of which many people are completely unaware.)

- Think of lengthening up the front of your body.

In fact, if you think or imagine any part of your body moving away from another part, it will encourage a release of muscle tension and help to improve your overall posture.

When Sir Winston Churchill said: 'There is nothing wrong with change, if it is in the right direction', I am pretty sure he was not thinking of the Alexander Technique, although it is perfectly apt for improving posture!

CHAPTER 12

Posture
and Shoes

The True Miracle.

The true miracle is not to fly in the air, or to walk on water, but to walk on this earth.

Chinese proverb

Many of us are prepared to suffer in the name of fashion, wearing clothing that is tight and uncomfortable, and restricts free movement, but the worst culprit of all in terms of posture is footwear. Have you ever wondered why we feel such relief when we kick our shoes off at the end of the day, or why we love walking barefoot along the beach, or why it is that many children love to go around barefoot? Perhaps our feet are trying to tell us something!

Each year, new types of shoe are designed and marketed, and we are promised that these will help us to 'walk the correct way', to 'burn fat as we walk' or that we will 'enjoy every step'. At the same time, more and more orthotics (shoe inserts) are being used to try to correct fallen arches, though in my experience the orthotics themselves can start to cause other postural problems that adversely affect the angle, knee or hip joints. Only recently I went into my daughter's class to give a talk about the Alexander Technique, and in a class of 30 children under the age of ten, 20 per cent of them were already wearing orthotics! The yearly rise in sales of orthotics indicates that something is terribly wrong with the way we are standing and walking.

In his article 'Why Shoes Make Normal Gait Impossible', podiatrist Dr William A Rossi claims that flaws in footwear affect the complex human function of walking. He argues that:

It took four million years to develop our unique human foot and our consequent distinctive form of gait, a remarkable feat of bioengineering. Yet, in only a few thousand years, and with one carelessly designed instrument, our shoes, we have warped the pure anatomical form of human gait, obstructing its engineering efficiency, afflicting it with strains and stresses and denying it its natural grace of form and ease of movement head to foot. We have converted a beautiful thoroughbred into a plodding plowhorse.

He argues that 'natural gait is biomechanically impossible for any shoe-wearing person... all shoes automatically convert the normal to the abnormal, the natural to the unnatural. And no therapy or mechanical device, no matter how precisely designed or expertly applied, can fully reverse the gait from wrong to right.'

Today, however, most people are not thinking about what shoes are doing to their posture because footwear has come to be associated with many symbolic values, and these can be the overriding factor when choosing a shoe. What used to be a simple, functional invention for protecting the foot has become a measuring stick of status, fashion and even self-esteem. People buy their shoes with the belief that these will help them to run faster, jump higher, prevent injuries, increase sex appeal and even earn them respect from others.

The human foot is often the only part of the human body that is in contact with the ground. It is a very complex and resilient structure: when we move as nature intended, the ankle serves as an amazing shock absorber, while the toes and reflexes act as a very efficient and effortless means of propulsion. The foot can sustain enormous pressure while remaining so flexible that we often refer to people as having a spring in their step when they walk. The foot and ankle contain 26 bones, which means that over a quarter of the bones in the human body are in the feet. Each foot contains 33 joints and more than 100 muscles, which adds to the amazing design, which is all too often taken for granted. All these components work together to provide the body with support, balance and mobility. By wearing inappropriate footwear, malfunctions can take place in the foot that can result in the development of problems elsewhere in the body. Similarly, abnormal tensions in other parts of the body can lead to problems in the feet.

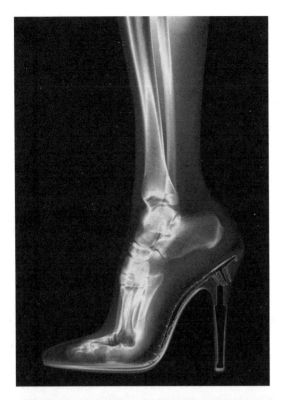

46: It took four million years to develop our unique human foot, yet the modern shoe can deform the foot and dramatically affect the way we walk. This can adversely affect the functioning of the rest of the body.

47: This is how the human foot is naturally designed to look... a long way away from the foot in photo 46!

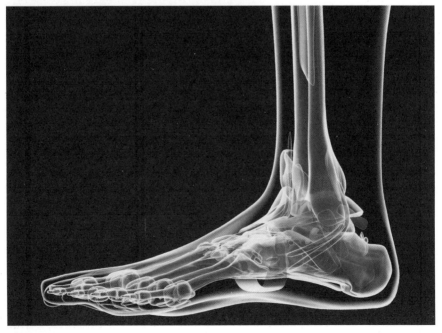

Millions of years of evolution have gone into the design of the human foot, yet many footwear designers all too often do not consider its wonderful design. Many shoe designers are primarily interested in how the shoes look and pay little attention to what shoes do to our feet and our posture. Most shoes that I have come across do not allow the foot to function as nature intended, and as a consequence they can adversely affect posture, balance and the way we move. Clearly something is not working, given the enormous sums of money spent on orthotics. The subject is vast and I could write a whole book on footwear, orthotics and walking, but let's explore the three most common problems with shoes.

Heels

The first problem is the height of the heel, or even the fact that there is a heel at all. I heard high-heeled shoes being discussed on a radio programme recently, and one woman was saying that when she was not able to wear her very high heels anymore because of back problems, she felt depressed, as though she was moving into a retirement home early. When barefoot, the body is naturally aligned, but even a low heel, such as those found in men's shoes, can contribute to the body being thrown out of alignment. According to Dr Rossi, if a person wears a 5cm (2in) heel, their entire body is thrown forward out of alignment by 20 degrees. In order to stop ourselves from falling forward, a huge number of changes must be made to the organization of our precisely balanced framework. The pelvis rotates forward, taking away support of the internal organs within the pelvic bowl and abdomen. The lumbar vertebrae become more arched as the body fights to regain balance, and as a consequence muscles, tendons and ligaments all become strained. Most importantly of all, being off balance cause a backward and downwards retraction of the head, causing excessive tension in the head, neck and back area, which will in turn interfere with the Primary Control, negatively affecting the functioning of the entire body. With each compensating adjustment, our structure moves away from the line of falling weight, greatly increasing the effort required to maintain an upright posture. When people wear higher heels, the problem obviously becomes much worse – the higher the heel, the more this tips the body forward, and the greater the misalignment caused. It is my personal view that although the occasional time when high heels are worn will not do any harm, the frequent use can add a great deal of unnecessary muscle tension throughout the body, which can adversely affect even the way we breathe.

The rigidity of the sole

The second problem is that the soles of many shoes are too stiff to allow much flexion. If they do flex, it is often in the wrong place, which is different from where the actual joints are. If you look at the design of the foot, you will easily see many joints in the toes, but most shoes bend in only one place, if at all. This can make many of the joints obsolete, and if a joint does not get used for long periods, it begins to malfunction. Some shoes are so rigid that they can also greatly restrict the range of natural movement of the arch of the foot, which can contribute to fallen arches.

❝ I was born with no natural aptitude. I wasn't pretty. I moved with no grace at all. I auditioned for the London Academy of Musical and Dramatic Arts but was not accepted. When I was finally admitted to Central School of Speech and Drama and showed up at my first movement class with my hump back and wearing a leotard, the movement teacher said, 'Oh God.' He sent me to the head of the school who then sent me to study the Alexander Technique with Dr Wilfred Barlow. That whole semester I took Alexander lessons instead of attending movement classes, which helped me enormously in my training and in subsequent years in my acting work. Now I can play people who are graceful and beautiful. ❞

Lynn Redgrave, actress

The space inside the shoe

Thirdly, shoes with a narrow fitting across the front of the foot prevent the natural weight-bearing expansion of the metatarsal bones. As a consequence, many people adopt a habit of walking with greatly reduced plantar flexion and start to take a step by sinking down onto the opposite hip socket. Compared to our natural gait, this is a fundamentally different way of walking that requires a great deal more muscular effort. It also changes the path of weight carried through the body and the sequence of weight distribution between foot and ground. In unrestricted walking, the pressure goes onto the front of the toes and pushes the toes apart, and activates one of the main postural reflexes called the plantar flexion reflex. When activated, it sends messages to the brain and spinal cord, which in turn trigger other postural reflexes. The lack of space in the front of the foot means the toes will become cramped and the postural reflexes are only partially triggered, and this can seriously affect the way we walk. We will then be forced to make further unnecessary effort just to take a step.

Natural walking and running

The way in which the weight is rolled across the sole of the foot while walking differs greatly between a person wearing shoes and one who is barefoot. When walking without shoes, the centre of the heel touches down first, the weight is then rapidly transferred through the lateral border to the ball of the foot. The heel then leaves the ground to prepare for the 'push-off', at which point we roll onto the big toe before taking a step. When walking in shoes, the pattern is different, and we can get clues from where the shoe is most worn on the inside. Often this is on the outside corner of the heel. This lopsided wear in concentrated areas indicates a loss of the natural way of standing, running and walking.

When running barefoot, our step sequence naturally changes to absorb the shock of ground impact. Instead of landing on the heels, it is the ball that makes first contact, thus using the arch of the foot as a shock-absorbing structure. Next the heel goes down momentarily, but does not necessarily reach the ground, before going back onto the balls and pushing off. In spite of this, the vast majority of recreational runners land heel first much more heavily than is healthy. This common mistake goes undetected because the cushioned soles of footwear mask the sensation of impact. So people unknowingly land too hard, and some runners are even instructed to put their heels down onto the ground, causing even greater impact. The shoe absorbs some of the impact, but not enough to completely protect the body, and over time this can cause problems. You can try this for yourself by doing the following exercise. First of all, run on the spot, making sure that your heels reach the ground. Do it slowly at first and then gradually increase the speed. It is easy to feel the impact throughout the whole body. Now do the same, but this time make sure you use the spring in your step by landing on your toes; make sure that the heel does not reach the ground. I'm sure you'll be able to feel an enormous difference.

A new shoe

During his teens and early twenties, my son, Tim, was a keen tennis player, and he developed a recurring ankle injury. While having Alexander Technique lessons with Colette Lyons in south-west England, Tim started to notice that some harmful habits he observed while walking, running and standing were partly caused by the shoes he was wearing. Colette, who originally trained as a physical education teacher, explained that some of Tim's problems were due to the inflexibility of his shoes, and during one of his lessons he realized that walking could be much less of an effort when making full use of the plantar flexion in the feet, as this encourages a greater spring in every step. Immediately after the lesson, however, when he began to walk home, he felt that the shoes he was wearing were once again detrimentally influencing his walking.

Over time, and with personal investigation, he found that the stiff soles and heels, the excessive cushioning, along with the heavy weight and narrow fit of his shoes were restricting the freedom of movement of both foot and ankle joints when running, walking and standing. He tried to find more flexible footwear, but realized that nearly all the shoes available were designed in a similar way.

The information he learned during his Alexander sessions became invaluable when he began studying product design at the Royal College of Art (London). For his final project he started to develop a new kind of footwear, keeping in mind what he had learnt during his Alexander

❝ The Alexander Technique has given me a greater awareness of the way my body moves and the way tensions move through my body. I have learned to release these tensions and to move more efficiently. It has helped me to play football with more confidence and has improved my coordination and balance. ❞

Andy Hunt, professional football player

Technique lessons. Using a back-to-basics philosophy, he started to design a shoe that was the closest thing to having bare feet while still providing adequate protection for the feet.

His studies required him to reinforce an experience-based philosophy with a good scientific grounding, and during his investigations he learnt that the first shoe was probably invented between 7,000 and 8,000 BC, not so much to safeguard feet from injury as he had thought, but to protect them from extremely cold temperatures. He also learned that in the US alone, 75 per cent of people suffer with foot problems of one kind or another, and as a consequence most people actually spend more on orthotics, foot surgery and other foot remedies than on actual shoes themselves! Of the five billion people who wear shoes around the world, 73 per cent of them have foot problems. Yet, in contrast, people who go barefoot in places like India, Africa and China are almost completely free from the foot problems that are so common in developed countries. He eventually designed a shoe that helped rather than hindered the natural way of walking. He called it the Vivo Barefoot Shoe.

Tim approached various shoe manufacturers, including members of the Clarks family, whose ancestors had created the famous Clarks Shoes company. They immediately saw the benefits and the potential of this new shoe and together they worked to bring the Vivo concept into production. Today, the shoe is sold all over the world under the name of Vivobarefoot, and production continues to increase as more and more people discover a shoe that is not only comfortable, but also good for their posture and health. Details of it can be found on page 179.

Using Vivobarefoot shoes, we naturally go up onto the balls of our feet, giving us excellent efficiency in locomotion in the same way as young children when they are just learning to walk. I have even come across people who claim that the shoes have brought their fallen arches back to life. Although I am really happy to be able to recommend Vivobarefoot shoes to people, it is important to point out that the shoes alone will not normally rid you of the tension you have accumulated throughout your life. However, the potent combination of Alexander Technique lessons and good footwear will be sure to help you to move through life with greater ease.

Albert Einstein once said: 'There are only two ways to live your life. One is though nothing is a miracle. The other is as though everything is a miracle.' If everything is a miracle, then human movement is one of the greatest and the less we interfere with that miracle the better.

CHAPTER 13

First Steps To Improving Posture

It is the body that is the hero, not antibiotics, nor machines or new devices. The task of the physician today is what it always has been, to help the body to do what it has learned so well to do on its own during its unending struggle for survival – to heal itself. It is the body, not medicine, that is the hero.

Dr Ronald J Glasser

Once you have started to take more time over your everyday activities, you will need to become aware of the unnecessary tension that you may be holding within your muscles. This tension is very likely to be impeding many of your movements, and it is not until you become aware of such tensions that you change anything. Alexander saw that many people were trying so hard to get good posture that they were practically paralysing the parts of the body that need to work. Self-awareness is the fundamental tool that will help you to become conscious of the postural habits that have arisen as a result of life's stresses and strains.

When I finally found a solution to my long-standing back problem, I could not understand why all the people who had tried to help me over the years had missed the obvious. It soon dawned on me that it was simply because they are not trained to do so. Their training involved learning about treatments intended to fix or alleviate symptoms, without first finding out why these had come about in the first place. Despite significant medical and scientific advances in recent years, the emphasis on treating symptoms rather than root causes is just as strong today. But knowledge of the Alexander Technique changes our expectations: in simple terms, why should we expect the medical profession to cure us of a problem that *we ourselves are causing*? We need to become aware of which muscles are over-tense and causing us to be pulled out of shape, with such painful consequences for us.

Alexander Technique lessons

The fastest, most efficient and effective way to do this is to have a course of Alexander lessons. I am sure I would never have worked out my problem without help. I know Alexander did, but it took him ten years, and required enormous patience, persistence and very creative thinking. It is generally easier to consult a trained teacher, much as we would when learning a musical instrument, horse-riding, driving, etc. So if we want to learn how to let go of the tension that is causing poor posture, it is very advantageous to go to an Alexander teacher. To my mind, to go to a doctor or other medical person and ask them to cure a problem that is directly caused by poor posture is like taking your car to a vegetable shop and asking them to fix your engine. But is the same the other way round: I would not have a clue how to help

“ Instead of feeling one's body an aggregation of ill-fitting parts, full of frictions and deadweights pulling this way and that so as to render mere existence in itself exhausting, the body becomes a coordinated and living whole, composed of well-fitting and truly articulated parts. It is the difference between chaos and order and so between illness and good health. ”

Sir Stafford Cripps, British Labour politician and Chancellor of the Exchequer (1947–50)

someone who had multiple injuries from a car accident, and I would be a fool to try.

Although it can be very helpful in the first instance to learn the principles and philosophy of the Alexander Technique from this book, it does not take the place of individual lessons, where a practical understanding of the Technique can be achieved. Each of us has a posture that is unique and therefore we have individual habits to recognize and let go of. The number of lessons needed will vary from person to person, depending on how ingrained their postural habits are and what they are hoping to achieve from the lessons. Many teachers recommend a course of between 20 and 30 lessons, but I personally believe that you can still learn a great deal about yourself in a basic course of as little as six to ten lessons. I always recommend a minimum of six lessons to give the person a chance to see the benefits. The Technique is not a 'quick fix' and it does take a few weeks to work, but the changes and benefits that occur are long-lasting. In my opinion, it is beneficial to have two lessons a week for the first two or three weeks. Later on, when you have grasped the principles of the Technique, you will be able to apply them on your own and you may find that a lesson once every two to three weeks is enough. Like any other subject, it is important to put into practice what you learn in a lesson in your everyday life.

What takes place during an Alexander lesson will vary depending on your own requirements and your teacher's teaching style. If the teacher has not been personally recommended to you, it might be worth having one lesson from two or three different teachers to see who suits you best. Various organizations will supply a list of qualified teachers (*see* pages on 179–80).

The Alexander 'experience'

The experience of the Alexander Technique can never be described in a book or conveyed in words. It is a wonderful feeling of lightness and ease that is brought about by all the parts of the body working in unison rather than in conflict. It gives many people a sense of peace and oneness that they had forgotten was possible, and some people describe this feeling as 'walking on air', or 'having well-oiled joints'. This feeling is natural: it is simply the feeling of letting yourself work as nature intended without any interference. Although the experience can differ from person to person, many feel a sense of lightness as they sit, stand and move, while others experience a sense of calmness or tranquillity, or feel as if their concerns and worries have been suddenly lifted from them. This feeling may last for only a short time after your first lesson, but with subsequent lessons the feeling of freedom, peace and ease will last for longer and longer periods of time as you learn to apply the Technique to all your daily activities. The Alexander Technique not only releases tension, but also redistributes the tension in the body, and you could describe it as a rebalancing of the entire system. Often, some muscles have become far too tense while others are not doing enough. During the process of learning the Technique, some muscles will become less tense while other muscles may in fact be required to do more work. Occasionally, after a lesson, people may feel an ache or discomfort in a different part of their body from the original problem area, but this is quite normal and will soon pass.

When you have learnt how to change the patterns of muscle tension, you will find that your posture has changed without any conscious effort on your part. This beneficial change in posture is bound to feel strange to begin with because we have become so accustomed to our poor posture over many years. It is similar to the experience of driving a different car than the one you are used to. Often the controls are in different places and you may have to push harder or less hard on the clutch and brake to operate them. However, if you drive this car for a week, it will begin to feel quite normal, and your own car may well feel a little strange when you drive it again. In the same way, you will need to give yourself time to get used to the new way of being, and after a few lessons you will become accustomed to the easier, freer way in which you sit, stand and move – and this will soon feel quite normal.

In all my 21 years of teaching, I have not come across one person who did not feel very odd when they first adopted new ways of sitting and standing. In fact, most people are amazed when I show them their new posture in a mirror at the end of their lesson as they are totally convinced that their shape is worse than before. They all have the impression that they are twisted or off balance, when they are really standing, sitting or moving with more grace and poise. This phenomenon is entirely due to the fact that many of us, like Alexander himself, are suffering from faulty sensory appreciation. It is impossible to rely on our kinaesthetic feelings (*see* page 102) because the very system that creates and evaluates these feelings is already going wrong. Because this is so common, Alexander often said to his pupils, 'Don't come to me unless, when I tell you you are wrong, you make up your mind to smile and be pleased.'

During a course of lessons, you will learn how to apply the Technique during your daily activities and be taught how to become aware of the excessive effort you are using. By changing the way we perform all our actions, we learn to move with greater ease and balance, and learn to prevent the tension from returning. This amounts to a re-education in which you learn new ways of walking, standing, sitting and bending that put less strain on you. If you have an occupation that is causing specific problems, like working at a computer, driving or playing a musical instrument, your teacher will go through those activities that may be causing the problems and show you how to perform them in a more conscious way that involves less effort. It is important to realize that you do not have to *do* anything to achieve a better posture or an improved way of using yourself while in activity. Learning how to do *less* leads to re-establishing harmony and ease in your life. This harmony and synchronization affect the mind and emotions too, and result in a more harmonious and conscious life. Ultimately, we need to stop being 'Human Doers' rather than Human Beings and start again to enjoy that deep part of ourselves that is still and present, and the Alexander Technique is a practical way to bring that still, alert consciousness – your 'Being' – back into everything we do.

The semi-supine position

This following procedure will help you to become more aware of the excessive muscular tension and you will begin to use thoughts (directions) to release some of that tension. Many people have found that this procedure can also be very successful in reducing stress, increasing vitality and reducing a wide variety of aches and pains. If it is done regularly, it can help to align the spine and improve your overall posture. For most people, the best time to do the lying down is in the morning, to get you observing your use of yourself before you start compressing your spine and tensing up. Second best is lunchtime, or mid-afternoon, but if you are at work or away from home, just do it as soon as you get back home. Some people who suffer with insomnia, however, find that they have an improved night's sleep if they lie in the semi-supine position just before going to bed, while others feel that

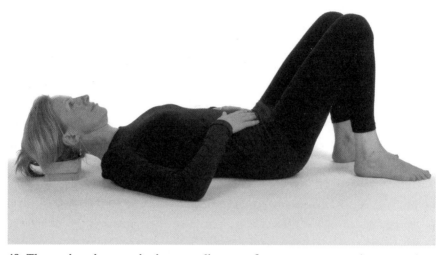

48: The semi-supine exercise is an excellent way for you to start to reduce muscular tension after a busy day.

starting the day in this way suits them better, and claim that they can feel the benefits throughout the rest of the day. Just do whatever works for you. Note, though, that it is better not to lie down after a heavy meal, as this will probably feel quite uncomfortable.

Lie down in the semi-supine position, as described below, initially for ten minutes each day, and lengthen the time progressively by adding one minute a day until you have reached 20 minutes. Remember, as I have said before, that real and lasting change does take time so perseverance and patience will be needed. Make notes each time you do it, as this will help you to see the changes. Never push yourself: it is not an endurance test. As you learn how to release tension, the lower back will gradually flatten on to the ground; this might take weeks or even months to happen, so please be patient with yourself. Make sure you do not push your back down onto the floor, as this will only make matters worse. Many of these tensions have taken years to accumulate so they are not going to disappear overnight. Some people say they do not have enough time to do this for the full 20 minutes in their busy working day; if this applies to you, just do it for whatever time you have. If for any reason you become uncomfortable, stop doing the exercise and consult your Alexander teacher.

The way to do the semi-supine exercise is simply to lie down on your back with some books underneath your head, your knees bent, your feet flat on the floor near to your pelvis without strain and your hands resting gently on either side of your navel or by your sides. Make sure you are lying on a carpeted floor and are warm enough, because it is much harder to release tension if you are feeling cold or lying in a draught. If necessary, place a blanket over yourself while you are lying down. The number of books beneath the head will vary from person to person, and it is better to use magazines or thin paperback books rather than hardbacks. If the books feel too hard, place a towel or some thin foam on top of the books. The best way to find out the right number of books is to ask your teacher when you start having Alexander lessons. If this is not possible for some reason, it is probably best to use a pillow or cushion until you can. As you are lying down, make sure that your head is not falling backwards or pushed too far forwards because it is crucial that your breathing and swallowing are unrestricted. The reason you have the books underneath your head is to give it support and to help combat the habit of pulling the head back, which can put pressure on the spine. Note, however, that it is still possible to pull your head back when you are simply lying there.

The soles of your feet should have an even contact with the ground and your knees need to be pointing towards the ceiling. Your feet should be near to your pelvis, but not so near that it is uncomfortable. If you find that your legs are falling in towards each other, or out away from each other, please follow one of these instructions, which will help to reduce muscle tension in the legs:

1. If the legs are falling *inwards* then move the feet *closer together.*

2. If the legs are falling *outwards* then move the feet *further apart.*

The back should be resting on the ground, but make sure you do not *do* anything in order to flatten it. One of the reasons that the knees are pointing to the ceiling is to enable the lower back to release onto the floor in comfort, but this may take some time.

At first, follow the same procedure as for the observation exercises on pages 131–33. Just be aware of any tension you can feel, making sure that you keep your eyes open throughout the exercise, as this will help you to stay focused.

Compare the left side of your body with the right to see if you feel symmetrical, but do not change anything. Now give yourself the following directions, which need to be repeated from time to time throughout the exercise:

- Allow your neck to be free.

- Think of your head going forward and up away from your spine.

- Allow your back to lengthen and widen onto the ground.

- Think of your shoulders widening away from one another.

- Think of your knees pointing up to the ceiling.

It is easier to let go of tension when lying down because gravity is working on your body in a different way and there are fewer balance issues and distractions to contend with.

This procedure is also known as 'active lying down', and although your body will be in a state of rest, it is not merely about resting, as you should be fully alert. If you find that your mind wanders off into other thoughts, try not to get annoyed with yourself, just bring your attention back gently to the present moment.

It is important to remember that you must not *do* anything or try to *find* the right position, as the emphasis for this exercise is on *doing less*. The directions listed above are just a few suggestions you can think about, but there are many more. Be creative and try to imagine others; as long as your thoughts involve allowing one part of the body to move away from another part, it will encourage a release of muscle tension. It may take a few days or even weeks before you feel totally comfortable with this new way of thinking, so please be patient.

In my first year of teaching the Alexander Technique, a man came to me who had been suffering from back pain for over 25 years. When I met him on his first lesson, he got a little notebook out of his top pocket and explained that he had spent over £87,000 trying to alleviate his back pain. For example, he had spent over £25,000 on operations and visits to the orthopaedic surgeons, another £15,000 on chiropractors, osteopaths and physiotherapists, a further £10,000 on complementary therapies and over £10,000 on back chairs that were sold to him on the basis that they would provide a

❝ The many obvious benefits that the technique afforded us as actors included minimized tension, centredness, vocal relaxation and responsiveness, mind/body connection and about an inch and a half of additional height. In addition, I have found in the ensuing years great benefits in my day to day living. By balancing and neutralizing tensions, I've learned to relieve as well as to avoid the aches and pains caused by the thousands of natural shocks that flesh is heir to. ❞

Kevin Kline, actor

solution to his pain, but actually did not help him. His travel bill came to a small fortune, as did all the gimmicks and gadgets he had purchased over the years, and he had kept a record of every penny he had spent.

On his first lesson, I showed him how to do the active lying down exercise and told him that he would need to do it every day for the next month. He became slightly agitated and asked me, 'Are you trying to tell me that I didn't need to spend the £87,000 on my back and that all I needed to do all along was your semi-supine exercise?' I thought for a moment and then said, 'Yes, that is what I am saying.' He became more agitated, even a little angry. I was unable to see him for two weeks after this lesson, as I was away on holiday, so when he returned for his second lesson he had been doing the lying down for a full three weeks. There was a visible change in him, and he seemed much more relaxed. He told me that he had not missed a day, and in fact on most days he had done the lying down twice, and since he had started he had had no pain whatsoever. After a few more lessons, his posture had completely changed and friends and relatives often commented on the visible difference in his posture. His story was quite exceptional, but it does illustrate the power of the semi-supine position.

Benefits of lying in the semi-supine position

Alexander teachers have observed that this activity:

- Improves overall posture.

- Allows the intervertebral discs to absorb fluid and helps to increase height.

- Helps to straighten the spine by helping to lessen the curves that have become exaggerated.

- Lengthens the spine so that it can support you better when you are upright.

- Releases muscular tension throughout your whole body.

- Improves your breathing by helping to release the intercostal muscles and the diaphragm.

- Improves circulation because the blood can flow better when the muscles are relaxed. Some of my pupils have found that their hands and feet have become warmer.

- Puts less pressure on the nerves that have become trapped due to over-tense muscles.

- Helps to prevent deterioration of the bones and joints of the spine and can even rejuvenate parts of the skeleton that have been worn from misuse of the body.

- Allows the internal organs to have more room to function.

- Helps to revitalize and re-energize you.

- Brings about an overall reduction in stress and tension physically, mentally and emotionally.

It is important to realize that these benefits will arise only if this exercise is done on a regular basis, once a day for at least ten minutes, and over a period of some weeks, though do not worry if you miss the odd day.

REMEMBER: At first you may not feel the changes that are happening, so be patient and do not try to force anything.

CHAPTER 14

Posture and Breathing

Breath is the bridge which connects life to consciousness, which unites your body to your thoughts.

Thich Nhat Hanh

Breathing is arguably the most important activity we will ever perform – it is the first thing we do as we come into the world and it is the last thing we will ever do as we leave. It quietly and consistently fills our lungs and gives us life. Its serene presence is always there, ready to be accessed at any moment, yet for the most part it goes unnoticed and unappreciated because we are preoccupied with other matters. The way we breathe can affect the way we live our lives – and the other way around. If we have a feeling of being rushed during our daily activities, our breathing often becomes faster and more shallow, so that we do not take in enough air. If we have a habit of breathing in a fast and shallow way, it's likely that we will feel that we are constantly in a hurry, never feeling we have enough time. It's easy to set up a vicious cycle where the quality of breathing deteriorates. These detrimental effects can often be seen in later life when people's breathing rate has become very rapid. If we are breathing naturally, on the other hand, we will feel generally more relaxed and more in control of our lives.

In natural circumstances, we take breaths without any effort on our part; we do not even have to remember to breathe, but we do need to learn how *not to interfere* with our primary life-enhancing mechanism. As you are reading these words, become aware of the silent inhalation and exhalation that is taking place at every moment. See if you can get a sense of the force or energy that is drawing the air into and then out of your lungs. As with many other natural functions of the body, many people unconsciously and habitually interfere with this simple act of breathing. The excessive muscular tension associated with poor posture can distort breathing, causing a lack of energy or tiredness. In extreme cases, misuse of the body can even exacerbate life-threatening breathing problems such as asthma.

To try to improve posture without reference to breathing, or to try to improve breathing without reference to posture, could be compared to talking about the act of eating without taking into account chewing. Posture and breathing are inseparable, and each one directly affects the other; the way we use ourselves, whether well or badly, will have an effect on how we breathe. It is easy to demonstrate this interrelatedness between posture and breath by sitting in a heavily slumped manner. If you try it for a moment or two (but not too long!), you can feel that you are unable to breathe deeply and freely. The same is true if you 'sit up straight' in a rigid way, by over-arching your back. If poor posture is a habit, then restricted breathing will also be a habit, leading to breathing problems. If we can learn to use ourselves in a more balanced way, our breathing will be less restricted, and if we learn to breathe well, it will help to reduce muscle tension so that we will be more able to sit, stand and move with poise and balance.

When Alexander began teaching the Technique, he was known as the 'breathing man' because he was able to help so many people improve the way they breathed. In fact, as we saw in earlier chapters, he developed the Technique to sort out his own breathing and voice problems, and he went on to use the Technique to help his fellow actors to improve theirs, through better posture, coordination and balance.

❝ The Alexander Technique has helped me to undo knots, unblock energy and deal with almost paralysing stage fright. ❞

William Hurt, actor

Over-tight muscles can affect the functioning of the ribcage, the lungs, and even the nasal passage, mouth and throat (trachea), through which air passes. They can also produce a general 'collapsing' or slumping of the whole torso, which can greatly restrict the lungs' capacity to take in air, leading to shallow breathing. Shallow breathing means that we have to expend more effort in order to take in sufficient air. In short, without realizing it, we can make the effortless act of breathing very hard work. This increased physical exertion goes largely unnoticed, because over many years we have become accustomed to our shallow and often laboured breathing, so that it just feels 'normal' and 'right' to us. A doctor once remarked that the average office worker does not take in enough air to keep a cat in good condition, and from my own experience I am inclined to agree with him. Many people do not know that their breathing patterns are poor, and sometimes the only time they experience the detrimental effects of poor breathing is when they exert themselves, such as when running for a bus or climbing a flight of stairs.

This pattern of interference with the respiratory system can sometimes be traced back as far as the age of five or six, because this is when many of us start to adopt a bent posture while bending over school desks. We learn to breathe badly when we are forced to hold these constricted positions for a great many hours during our developing years. The poor posture that most of us developed from hunching over school desks not only causes graceless, uncoordinated or even clumsy movements, but also restricts our breathing, causing us to take in less air than is good for us.

Many of our detrimental respiratory habits may go unnoticed during childhood or adolescence, but the evidence of fast, shallow breathing can more easily be seen in adulthood as it becomes more ingrained and accentuated. In severe cases, it is possible to observe adults unnecessarily raising and lowering their shoulders while inhaling and exhaling, directly due to excessive tension around the ribcage. Others hold their abdominal muscles rigid and then lift and collapse the chest in order to breathe, because they are trying to sit up very straight or wrongly think that they should have a flat stomach. If we are unable to get enough oxygen because of unnatural interference in the workings of the respiratory system, we will unconsciously try to find another way of achieving a greater intake of oxygen. This is done by increasing the breathing rate, which results in a quicker, more shallow pattern of respiration.

By comparison, if you observe a baby or young child, you may notice how much the abdomen and ribcage move in and out rhythmically with each breath. The rest of the body remains in a state of relaxation while the air is taken in and expelled almost effortlessly. In fact, it seems like the whole body is breathing.

Stress and breathing

The way we breathe affects our state of mind, energy level, the way we feel emotionally and even the way we move. In the short term, a fast, shallow type of breathing does not cause harm, but in the long term habitually shallow or fast breathing can cause or exacerbate negative states of mind such as anxiety, worry, panic attacks and general stress. Any one of these conditions can in turn cause further interference of the breathing mechanism, and a vicious circle is created. If someone is anxious in a situation that requires calm and collected thought, we often tell them to 'take a deep breath' as a way of calming down. In the same way, by bringing our attention to the way we breathe, we can begin to become aware of and change the detrimental habits that interfere with this delicate process. By relearning our natural rhythm of breathing, we can alter the way we think, feel and act while carrying out our everyday activities.

When most people come for Alexander lessons, they do not specifically complain of breathing problems, and, if asked, they will say that their breathing is fine. However, I find that many people are breathing too fast, too shallowly or in an erratic manner; often they do not even give themselves time to finish one breath before they start the next. This is a direct reflection of how they have been living their lives, and they will frequently say that they feel that there are never enough hours in a day. This fast pace of life in which many people feel they are caught up causes over-tensing of many muscles and the associated restrictive breathing pattern, which causes harm to their physical health, their state of mind and their quality of life. After a course of Alexander lessons, I find that a person's breathing rate usually decreases naturally, often by up to a third.

Breathing exercises

Today there are many schools of thought on how to improve breathing, but many of these ways involve some kind of breathing exercise, which in many cases unfortunately only encourages more bad habits and can do more harm than good. With all good intentions, many voice trainers and physical educators encourage 'deep breathing' as a way of getting the lungs to work more efficiently, and while their aim may be sound in principle, the way in which they encourage their students to achieve this may actually exacerbate many respiratory problems. People are often instructed to increase their lung capacity by 'pulling in' or 'pushing out' their breath, but this creates further pressure on an already overstrained muscular system. Breathing exercises commonly focus on the in-breath, as, for example, the instruction to 'take a deep breath', but this will invariably cause the person to tighten muscles and increase the interference with the entire breathing mechanism. Tightening and shortening the muscles can result in arching of the back and lifting of the chest, which causes additional faulty breathing patterns and makes the original breathing habits even more deeply ingrained.

In contrast, the Alexander Technique encourages more natural breathing by a process of *unlearning* detrimental habits, rather than practising specific breathing exercises. The late Dr Wilfred Barlow, an Alexander teacher and consultant rheumatologist working in the National Health Service in the UK, was convinced that the person suffering from asthma needed 'breathing education' rather than a set of exercises. In his book *The Alexander Principle,* he wrote: 'The asthmatic needs to be taught how to stop his wrong way of breathing. Breathing exercises have, of course, frequently been given by physiotherapists for this and for other breathing conditions, but the fact is that breathing exercises do not help the asthmatic greatly – in fact, recent studies show that after a course of "breathing exercises", the majority of people breathe less efficiently than they did before they started them.... the asthmatic does not need breathing exercises – he needs breathing education. He needs a minute analysis of his faulty breathing habits and clear instructions on how to replace them by an improved use of his chest.'

Over the last 20 years, many asthma sufferers have come to me for help with breathing and I have found that they can learn to breathe more freely by improving their overall posture. Due to the benefits of the Technique, many have dramatically reduced or stopped their medication (while under their doctor's supervision).

How breathing works

Without making it too complex, it might be helpful to have a basic understanding about how the respiratory system works. The lungs are among the biggest organs in the body. Our total lung capacity ranges from 4 to 6 litres (7 to 10½ pints), and we breathe approximately 11,000 litres (2,420 gallons) of air in any one day. The lungs are enclosed within a mobile ribcage: the very top of the lung is actually situated above the collarbone and the bottom of the lung extends almost to the bottom of the ribcage (*See* photo 49). Just below the lungs is a very powerful muscle called the diaphragm, which is crucially involved in the process of breathing. It is a large dome-shaped muscle that is attached to the lowest ribs.

When you breathe in:
The diaphragm contracts, causing it to lose its 'dome' shape as it moves downwards and flattens out, making the area within the ribcage expand. At the same time the lower ribs move outwards. These actions allow more room in the thoracic cavity, so that the lungs have a greater capacity to receive air. When the diaphragm is stretched to a certain point, a 'stretch reflex' is triggered and it, *automatically and without us having to do anything,* starts to return to its original dome shape.

When you breathe out:
The exact opposite happens: the diaphragm relaxes and returns to its dome shape, causing the capacity within the ribcage to decrease. The sternum drops and the lower ribs move inwards. This has an overall effect of reducing the area in the thoracic cavity and causes the lungs to expel air. As we exhale, the air pressure in the lungs decreases, creating a partial vacuum, which then causes the air from outside to be sucked into our lungs *automatically and without us having to do anything.* This causes the diaphragm to contract, and it starts to move downwards once again, thus completing a natural cycle. Under normal conditions, the entire breathing mechanism should be self-governing and therefore is sometimes referred to as working 'automatically'. Contrary to what many people think, it is the out-breath, rather than the in-breath, that determines the way we breathe, yet many exercises focus on 'taking an in-breath' rather than allowing more air to be released. In fact, the more air we exhale, the deeper the next inhalation will

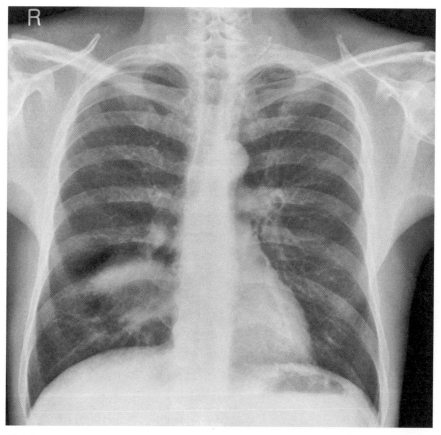

49: The lungs, as shown as darker area, are much bigger than many people think. They extend from above the collarbone to almost the bottom of the ribs.

be, and the deeper our breathing will become. So the first thing you need to do to improve your breathing is to allow yourself to finish one breath before you start to breathe in. It is important to remember that you should not force the air out, because this also causes excessive tension and interferes with natural breathing.

Improving breathing

Alexander was a trained reciter, and efficient breathing was essential to his skilful recitation. He helped people to breathe more easily during their lessons with him. He was famously quoted as saying: 'I see at last that if I don't breathe... I breathe', because his Technique is based on 'doing less' –

that is, instead of willing oneself to breathe in a certain way, the key is rather to stop interfering with the natural breathing process, so that it can happen naturally by itself. Relearning how to breathe freely can be very beneficial to public speakers or indeed anyone involved in the performing arts, because many speakers, actors and musicians become nervous before or during a presentation, concert or performance, and nervous tension can adversely affect the way they perform, in extreme cases even preventing them from performing altogether. By ensuring that we breathe naturally, we can effectively combat the effects of stress. In this way, we will feel calmer and more in control even at times of intense emotional or mental stress.

Just by focusing your attention on how you breathe without trying to change it, you can bring about an improvement. Take a moment and begin to be aware of your breathing as you are standing or sitting. Ask yourself the following questions:

- How rapid is my breathing?

- How deeply do I breathe?

- Are my ribs moving as I breathe?

- If so, which part of the ribcage is moving most?

- How much movement is there in the abdominal region when I breathe?

- Do I feel any restriction in my breathing, and if so, where?

It is crucial that you do not deliberately alter the way you breathe; just simply become aware of the inhalation and the exhalation, as this is often enough to bring about a favourable change. Becoming aware of tension is the first step in learning how to breathe more naturally.

To help his pupils relearn how to breathe naturally, Alexander developed the following method, which is known as the 'whispered ah' procedure. He always maintained that he did not like using exercises as they could encourage habits and could have the effect of stopping people thinking for themselves, so he developed the following procedure and maintained that it was essentially an exercise in inhibition and to prevent 'end-gaining' while breathing.

The 'Whispered ah' Procedure

1. First of all, take a moment use your directions as set down earlier in the book.

2. Notice where your tongue is and let it rest on the floor of the mouth with the tip lightly touching your lower front teeth. This allows for a free passage of air to and from the lungs.

3. Think of something amusing that makes you smile, because that mental act lifts the soft palate, which helps to create an unrestricted passage for the air to flow freely. It also can help your lips and facial muscles to release tension.

4. Gently *and without straining*, let your lower jaw drop so that your mouth is open. If you allow gravity to do most of the work, your head will not tilt backwards in the process.

5. *Whisper* an 'ah' sound (as in the word 'laughter') until you come to the natural end of the breath. It is important not to rush the procedure by forcing the air out too quickly or trying to empty the lungs by extending the 'ah' sound as long as possible. Gently close your lips and *allow* the air to come in through your nose and fill up your lungs.

6. Notice if you have tightened in some areas while whispering the 'ah'.

7. Repeat this procedure several times.

Be aware of your breath as it travels in through your nose, down your throat and into your lungs. Just being conscious of your breathing will bring about subtle changes of which you may not even be aware. Again, it is important to remember that *trying* to change your breathing in any way will interfere with the body's natural processes. You may also like to use other whispered sounds, like 'ee', 'oo' or 'sss', and you can vocalize these sounds too. On inhalation, the air has to travel *horizontally* through your nose – many people think that the air direction is *up* the nose, but examination of the bones of the skull shows that the nasal passage is in fact a horizontal opening.

You can try this for yourself. Take a deep breath, imagining the air travelling *up* your nose, and now do the same but imagining the air travelling *horizontally through* your nose. You will probably find the second breath takes much less effort. Some people also find it helpful to imagine breathing in through the eyes, as this can help prevent tightening of the neck or throat muscles during the 'whispered ah' procedure.

Regular practice of the 'whispered ah' can help you to free yourself from harmful breathing habits and can, over time, help you to develop a more efficient respiratory system. Once again, it is strongly recommended that initially you go through this routine with your Alexander teacher, as it is easy to misinterpret the instructions. Also, due to *faulty sensory appreciation* it is often the case that we maybe tensing our muscles unconsciously. In other words, when we are following these instructions we may be doing something else without realizing it. For example, it is very common for people to pull the head back onto the spine instead of just allowing the jaw to drop while carrying out the third instruction, while others are convinced that they are opening their mouth wide when there is actually a gap of less than 2cm (³/₄ in) between their upper and lower lips. If for any reason you are unable to have lessons (for instance, because there is no teacher near you), then it is important to perform the 'whispered ah' in front of a set of mirrors, as this will give you a better idea of whether or not you are carrying out the instructions correctly. Remember: natural breathing is an involuntary process, and when we don't interfere with it, breathing will take care of itself.

Posture and the voice

Many people are unaware that speaking and singing involve the whole self, and both of these activities are adversely affected by poor posture. If we want to learn to speak or sing effectively and confidently, we first need to be sure to eliminate the voice's most powerful obstacle, namely muscle tension. To ensure that our voices are being produced in the most effective and efficient manner, the first thing we need to consider is the way we are using ourselves during the activity.

The way we breathe during all acts of voice production, including conversational speaking, is of paramount importance. The lungs act like bellows, forcing air up through the larynx, where the vocal cords are located, causing them to vibrate. This sound is then amplified in the cavities of the head, and the tongue, the palate, teeth and lips articulate and impose consonants and vowels on the amplified sound. This sound will be affected if the body is being pulled out of alignment due to excessive tension in the muscles. Try making a vocalized 'ah' sound, then drop your head before pulling it back onto your spine and you will see that your voice changes significantly. In this way you can see that even the way we speak is affected by our posture.

The enjoyment of breathing

Natural breathing is not only an essential part of existence – it can also be one of life's great joys. It can be a pure pleasure to feel the air filling you with life and offering you the gift of yet another moment to appreciate its wonders. The Italian poet and novelist Giovanni Papini once said that breathing is the greatest pleasure in life. Being aware of your breathing and practising the 'whispered ah' regularly can be a powerful way to calm your entire system and allow you to be in the present moment to experience the true miracle of being alive.

By *allowing* your breathing to return to its natural rhythm, it will become deeper and freer, and your body will start to function more efficiently. Many people feel 'energized' with a renewed enthusiasm for life as they feel the power of their spirit flowing through them. With every breath comes another opportunity to throw away the habits that bind us so tightly, so that we can start to make real choices in our lives. Through free choice we have the power to turn life into what we want it to be, rather than spending it constantly chasing endless goals. So perhaps these wise words of Thich Nhat Hanh can do wonders for your posture: 'Smile, breathe and go slowly.'

CHAPTER 15

Bringing Your Life Back Into Balance

Beyond all rights and wrongs, there is a field –
I will meet you there.

Rumi

I hope it has been clear that the issue of posture is not merely physical, but goes to the very core of our being. It affects our health, our emotions and our attitude to life. Your posture is a direct reflection of who you are, or at least who you perceive yourself to be, and without a doubt it can directly affect how others see and treat you. Your posture is an integral part of who you are, so by changing your posture for the better, you will not only change the way you sit, stand and move, but also enhance the way you think and feel. In turn when you are able to think more clearly and feel calmer, you will inevitably have better posture. As we have seen, poor posture is not just something that happens to you; it is actually the consequence of the way you have been using yourself in all your actions. By learning and applying principles of the Alexander Technique and implementing the suggestions in this book, you will slowly but surely start to feel more balanced, coordinated and integrated, and this will help you to feel at ease with yourself and others.

Many other aspects of your life can come back into balance. Improving posture is not only good for your health; but also beneficial for your social life, your working life, your relationships with others and, indeed the whole of your life. Robert Louis Stevenson once said: 'To be what we are and to become what we are capable of becoming is the only end of life'; many of us however have yet to discover what our hidden potential really is. Because improving posture can increases inner confidence, this can help us to explore our creative talents – some that may have been suppressed for many years and others that we may have never used.

To really improve your posture on a deep level you will need to move away from the idea of trying to adopt a particular way of positioning yourself while sitting or standing and realize that the effects of posture, whether good or bad, pervade the whole self, being inextricably bound up in everything you do or say. It is present when you greet somebody new, or tie up your shoes, or even in the way you bring a glass up to your lips. It is the accumulation of the way you use yourself in all things. Posture is part of the way we think, our attitude to life and how we react emotionally to other people. The only effective and lasting way that we can change our posture is to change the way we use ourselves, physically, mentally and emotionally, as it is by changing our thoughts and attitudes that we really bring about change in the way we live.

Posture and emotions

Alexander once said that we translate everything, whether physical, mental or spiritual, into muscular tension. In other words, past traumas and unexpressed feelings can be trapped within the muscles and culminate in the fixed posture that we have adopted. Some of these habits can originate from before we could talk and therefore feel a part of who we are. Without our realizing it, these suppressed unconscious feelings can result in habitual reactions that are running our lives and our relationships with others. Sometimes certain things that people say or do can 'trigger' past feelings that are totally out of proportion to the present incident, and our reactions can result in further muscle tension, which only compounds the problem. Even when we are not reacting in certain situations, these outworn mental and emotional ways of protecting ourselves can be physically held in the body in the form of excessive muscle tension, eventually turning into such strong habits that they can dramatically affect our posture. As a result, other systems (like the respiratory or circulatory systems) within the body will have to work much harder because of the huge pressures and limitations exerted on the internal organs, muscles and joints. Eventually the body may lose the ability to function normally, resulting in illnesses.

You do not necessarily have to enter into years of therapy in order to change your behaviour; simply learning to inhibit the automatic habitual reaction before you act can change a great deal about the way you think and behave during your daily activities. Aristotle is reported to have said: 'Anyone can become angry – that is easy. But to be angry with the right person, to the right degree, at the right time, for the right purpose, and in the right way – that is not easy.' By using inhibition, you can bring under control many of the emotions that may have become out of balance and learn a new *constructive conscious control* of yourself. Through consciously choosing to release the muscular tension that has formed due to suppressed emotions, rigid thought patterns and fixed prejudices, you can live a happier, more harmonious life.

As you have seen, trying to change one's posture by merely altering one's body position really achieves nothing of any lasting benefit, and in some cases can actually make matters worse. However, to bring awareness to how we sit, stand and move, and then to decide to move with consciousness and deliberateness, can speak volumes about who we are. There is, in fact, no one right posture – any position is a valid position; poor posture is merely a habitual tendency that is often inappropriate for the task at hand. No one position will cause you harm if done once in a while; it is the subconscious stereotyped behaviour patterns – your postural habits – that you repeat hundreds of times a day without knowing it, that cause many of your postural problems. Often children will walk around a playground on tiptoe or walk on their heels, and as it is done consciously (i.e. it is not habitual), it does not cause a problem. If, however, they did either of these actions habitually, it would obviously result in some leg or foot problems in the longer term.

When changing our posture on a deep level, we are not really learning anything new, but rather rediscovering something very old. Almost every one of us had beautiful graceful posture when we were small, and by using the Alexander Technique we can rediscover that this free and aligned posture is still within us, although it may have been dormant for many years or even decades. Improving posture really means bringing our habits to conscious awareness and deliberately choosing to replace those that are no longer serving us with new ways of responding that are more beneficial and natural. Alexander once said: 'When an investigation comes to be made, it will be found that every single thing we are doing in the Work [the Technique] is

❝ I had chronic back trouble for up to 20 years which was related to a football injury. Often my back would go into spasm, which would put me in serious pain. I tried everything from acupuncture to chiropractic. I even had surgery, which involved the removal of two discs but this was never completely satisfactory. Then I went to an Alexander Technique teacher. He taught me how to walk correctly and how to sit down correctly. He explained to me about the weight of my head on my body and made me aware of the importance of good posture and how to have conscious control of it. … Of all the therapies I tried, none of them has been as good as the Alexander Technique. ❞

Eamon Dunphy, former Irish international football player and sports journalist

exactly what is being done in nature where the conditions are right, the difference being that we are learning to do it consciously.'

Being present

The first and most important habit to change if we are ever going to make progress is the tendency not to be truly present while we go about our daily activities. This is a habit that prevents us from being in the here and now, and unless we are conscious in the present moment, how will we ever be able to be aware of what we are doing? Alexander called the habit of not being in the here and now 'mind-wandering', and once we start to practise being more present, our posture will invariably start to change. Notice young children who have beautiful posture – they are completely focused on what they are doing, and we can do the same. It just takes a little practice.

The psychologist and spiritual teacher Dr Richard Alpert (Ram Dass),

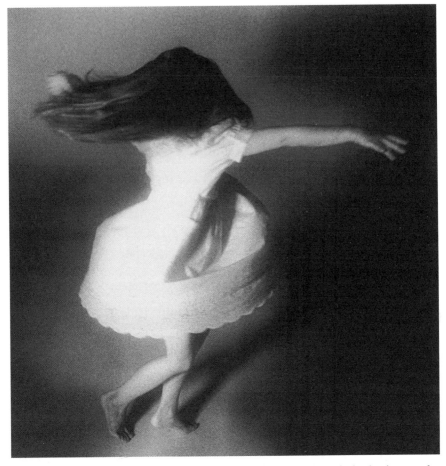

50: Having good posture is enjoyable, flowing and relaxed; it includes having good balance, poise, awareness, grace of movement, free thinking and free emotions.

author of *Be Here Now*, often talks of 'Somebody Training', which he says begins at a very early age. We all came into the world with an open mind, an open heart and a free body – as small children, our thoughts, actions and emotions were pure and uncomplicated, and we did not have concepts of what we should do, say or feel. However, as we grew up, our parents and teachers wanted us to grow up to be somebody special, and they set about training us to really be 'somebody'. They may not have realized that we were already special just the way we were, and they set about teaching us what to say and do. We were even instructed as to what we should be feeling and how we should express ourselves. This 'somebody training', which takes place over many years, is often based on the values and ideals that our family and teachers themselves were taught when they were growing up. After this 'indoctrination, socialization and child development programme' we unsurprisingly often end up ourselves wanting to be 'somebody special'. The only trouble is that the 'somebody' we end up being is not usually the person we really are, as it is based on someone else's concepts and theories. Along with this artificial personality comes an artificial posture, because our posture is really a compilation of fixed thought patterns and false ways of being that we have been taught, and is not really us. The main problem is that we do not realize it, but all we know is that we may feel unfulfilled in our work, in our relationships and in our lives in general. It is interesting to realize that many people aspire to be more sophisticated, yet the very word 'sophisticated' means 'to be false, no longer simple or natural'. So in reality the unnatural posture that many of us have adopted is also our prison. It was created by the indoctrination that planted in us erroneous ideas about who we really are.

The story of Zumbach the tailor illustrates this well. A man went to buy a suit for his wedding and, wanting only the very best, he ordered his suit from the most expensive and reputable tailor in town. The tailor's name was Zumbach and he took hours meticulously measuring and remeasuring. The suit took many weeks to make and finally the day arrived when it was ready. The man happily made his way down to the tailor's shop, only to find that the suit did not fit at all. Angrily, he called Zumbach and said, 'There is something wrong with this suit! One sleeve is much shorter than the other!' 'There is nothing wrong with the suit,' Zumbach replied, 'it is just the way that you are standing.' Zumbach then adjusted the posture of the man, pushing his shoulder right down and said, 'If you stand like this, the suit will fit perfectly.' The man was still not convinced and said, 'But what about the bulge in the back of the neck, surely that should not be there on such an expensive suit?'

Zumbach grew impatient. 'Sir, I assure you the suit is perfect... it is merely the way you are holding yourself. If you pull your other shoulder up and drop your head down, then the suit will fit perfectly.' After a few more alterations in his posture, the man left the shop and was walking down the road when a woman came running up to him and exclaimed, 'What a beautiful suit you have, I bet Zumbach the tailor made it for you.' 'How did you know that?' the man asked. 'Only a tailor with the special talent of

Zumbach could make a suit to fit a person as bent and twisted as you are!', replied the woman.

In the same way, throughout our lives many of us have adopted various postures as a reaction to certain stimuli or to suit the situations that we have found ourselves in. Perhaps an emotional reason such as shyness or a lack of self-esteem caused us to hunch our shoulders or tense our joints or maybe many hours spent sitting in a car or behind a desk caused a bent spine, but whatever the reason for our poor posture, it can change for the better. Through this process of changing your posture, not only will you be improving the way you look, healing a back or neck problem, or even improving your breathing or voice, you will also be improving the way you think, feel and act. So while it is true that the Alexander Technique has helped many people with a wide variety of health issues, it also has a much deeper purpose: its true power lies in breaking through the facade about who you think you are and helping you to rediscover who you really are. If used at its deepest level, the Technique can help to free you from your past conditioning and the erroneous ideas that you may have about yourself. It has the power to enable you to be the free and creative person that you really are. Even having the desire to improve your posture is an indication that you want to embark on the journey towards true freedom. Remember, though, that the change will happen slowly, so don't be in any hurry, because it is in hurrying that we start to lose our sense of ourselves once again.

A philosophy for living

As you take the steps needed to improve the way you use yourself, you will find that you not only are more conscious of how you sit, stand and move, but also become much more aware of the world about you, as your senses of sight, hearing, touch, taste, smell and balance are heightened. You will eventually find that pausing before acting becomes natural and normal rather than unusual, and this will enable you to have a greater choice as you go about your daily activities. Many people find that as they improve their posture through the Alexander Technique, they find a practical philosophy for living and as a result feel more alive. In the *Tao Te Ching* it says: 'When you let go of what you are, you become what you might be; when you let go of what you have, you receive what you need.' Have you ever struggled to achieve a goal, only to find that after you have given up, the goal is accomplished without you even trying? In a way it is the same with posture – once you stop *trying* to improve your posture and just let go of your tensions, your habits and your thoughts, a new way of being will automatically materialize. This change occurs on all levels. For example, people who have always disliked their work suddenly find the confidence to pursue a career that they have always wanted to have, while others decide to do something they have always wanted to do but never allowed themselves. Improved posture often gives people improved confidence and self-esteem.

I would like to finish with a quotation from *A New Earth* by Eckhart Tolle:

> You are a human being. What does that mean? Mastery of life is not a question of control, but of finding a balance between human and Being.
>
> Mother, father, husband, wife, young, old, the roles you play, the functions you fulfil, whatever you do – all that belongs to the human dimension.
>
> It has its place and needs to be honoured, but in itself it is not enough for a fulfilled, truly meaningful relationship or life.
>
> Human alone is never enough, no matter how hard you try or what you achieve.
>
> Then there is Being.
>
> It is found in the still, alert presence of Consciousness itself,
>
> The Consciousness that you are.
>
> Human is form. Being is formless.
>
> Human and Being are not separate but interwoven.

The Alexander Technique is a very practical way to put the 'Being' back into everything that you 'do', and by accomplishing this you can truly enter the magical realm of the present moment, which in reality is the only place in which everyone and everything exists. By doing so you will recognize how special you really are. You will be able to prevent the fear of the future or the regrets of the past dominating your life and there will no longer be a need to hide from your fellow human beings. Your new state of being will naturally be reflected in your posture, which will become open, upright and poised without any effort. By improving posture, you will not only improve your physical stance and movements, but you can also rediscover the true magic of what it means to be a living, free and magnificent being. The only thing that you will be required to do is to let go of the habits that hold you back, so that you can come into the present moment and enjoy this incredible journey of self-discovery though conscious choice.

❝ The Alexander Technique really works. I recommend it enthusiastically to anyone who has neck pains or back pain. I speak from experience. ❞

Roald Dahl, author of many children's books

Appendix

Randomized controlled trial of Alexander Technique lessons, exercise and massage (ATEAM) for chronic and recurrent back pain

During the period between November 2001 and August 2008 a major randomized controlled clinical trial, funded by the Medical Research Council and the NHS, was carried out in the UK. It clearly showed that Alexander Technique lessons give long-term benefit to chronic low-back pain sufferers. This multicentre trial involving 579 patients, led by GP researcher Professor Paul Little, University of Southampton, and GP Professor Debbie Sharp, Bristol University, is one of the few major studies to show significant long-term benefits for patients with chronic low-back pain. The trial assessed the benefits provided by Alexander Technique lessons, classical massage and normal GP care. Half the patients allocated to each intervention also received a GP prescription for general aerobic exercise.

The conclusions of the trial were that one-to-one lessons in the Alexander Technique from registered teachers have long-term benefits for patients with chronic back pain. These findings have led to improved understanding and acceptance of the Technique by the medical profession in recent years and an increase in the number of doctors referring patients for Alexander Technique lessons.

Comment from a GP
'From a discal neck injury in 1990 I developed progressive spinal problems. By 2002 I had suffered mechanical neck and back pain, several episodes of nerve root pain at different levels with loss of power and reflexes in my arms. I saw four neurosurgeons, who all recommended different neck operations. I then developed complex regional pain syndrome and could barely use my right arm. I was in unbearable pain and virtually unable to move my neck. I started taking

Alexander Technique lessons and began to experience improvement and lessening of pain after some 12 to 15 lessons. I did regular Alexander Technique for about four years. I have had progressive improvement since 2003 such that I now have no neck or arm pain. Alexander Technique lessons from a good teacher are an effective technique and were instrumental in my recovery. Based on simple applied principles it can afford sustained relief from pain of spinal origin. It teaches the body to undo neuromuscular tensions and reduce strain in normal motor function; probably cost effective were it taught in primary health care. I welcome this positive trial evidence.'

Dr Nick Mann GP

Full trial details can be seen on the British Medical Journal website: www.bmj.com/content/337/bmj.a884.full

Understanding the Terminology

Being present/attentive Being in the present moment and focusing your attention on the activity you are performing; not letting your mind wander into the past or future.

Conscious control The main aim of learning and applying the Alexander Technique: it is a state of being where you are using awareness and free choice to make clear informed decisions about your actions, rather than reacting in a stereotyped, habitual way.

Direction A mental order that your mind gives to the body.

End-gaining Being too goal-oriented: thinking only of the end and not giving any consideration to the way in which you achieve the goal.

Faulty sensory appreciation Thinking or sensing you are doing one thing when in fact you are doing something completely different, such as feeling that you are standing up straight when in fact you are leaning backwards.

Fear reflex Alexander used this term to describe the body's reaction to any stimulus that causes fear. Any fearful conditions can cause excessive muscular tension, which, if they happen frequently, can start to develop into a habit. A good example of this is the over-contraction of neck muscles, which can continuously pull the head back onto the spine, causing neck and back problems.

Free choice To become aware of unconscious habits and choose a different reaction to your habitual one.

Habit/habitual actions Any action or thought that we feel is difficult not to do or think; often habits are below the level of consciousness and therefore we are completely unaware of them.

Inhibition The act of refraining from a habit or reaction and choosing a different response.

Kinaesthetic sense The sense that informs you where your body is in space at any given time; the brain detects movements of the muscles and senses any movement you are making.

Means whereby Paying attention to the action you are doing, which involves inhibition and direction; working out in advance how you are going to go about your activity.

Mind-wandering Allowing your thoughts to move away from the present moment; not paying attention.

Posture All aspects of how you use yourself; not only just physical but mentally and emotionally, too.

Primary Control A dynamic relationship between the head, neck and the rest of the body, which helps to coordinate movement and posture harmoniously.

Psycho-physical unity The mind, emotions and the body acting as one unit: they are not separate entities, but merely different facets of the Self.

Self The entire Human Being – including everything mental, physical, emotional and spiritual – which is whole and indivisible.

Tension Unnecessary muscular activity – we obviously need a certain amount, but many people have far too much for a healthy life.

Thinking in activity Using inhibition and direction while performing any action.

Use More than just posture: it is the way or ways in which we carry out all our activities, physical, mental and emotional.

Resources

Useful Websites

Richard Brennan's websites with useful articles and information about the Alexander Technique www.alexander.ie or www.alexandertechniqueireland.com

Details of good-quality **wedge cushions** and chairs that improve posture www.alexander.ie/shop.html

Details of **footwear** designed with the Alexander Technique in mind www.vivobarefoot.com or www.terraplana.com/vivobarefoot_benefits.php

Website of *Direction Journal* – a wonderful magazine publishing articles and information for teachers and students of the Alexander Technique. Visit the website for free audios, articles, live interviews plus 25 years of back issues in stock! www.directionjournal.com

The International Societies of Teachers of the Alexander Technique below give details of how to find a teacher nearest to you. All teachers listed on these websites have undergone extensive three-year training.

UK
Website for teachers in the Society of Teachers of the Alexander Technique (STAT), the first and longest-established Alexander Technique organization. Teachers listed are mainly from the UK and Ireland, but also include many other countries.
www.stat.org.uk

AUSTRALIA
Australian Society of Teachers of the Alexander Technique (AuSTAT)
www.austat.org.au

BELGIUM
Belgian Association of Teachers of the Alexander Technique (AEFMAT)
www.fmalexandertech.be

BRAZIL
Associaçáo Brasileira de Técnica Alexander (ABTA)
http://abtalexander.com.br

CANADA
Canadian Society of Teachers of the F. M. Alexander Technique/Société Canadienne des Professeurs de la Technique F. M. Alexander (CanSTAT)
www.canstat.ca

DENMARK
Dansk forening af lærere i Alexanderteknik (DFLAT)
www.dflat.dk

FINLAND
Suomen Alexander-tekniikan Opettajat (FINSTAT)
www.finstat.fi

FRANCE
L'Association Française des Professeurs de La Technique Alexander (APTA)
www.techniquealexander.info

GERMANY
Alexander Technik Verband Deutschland (ATVD)
www.alexander-technik.org

IRELAND/EIRE
The Irish Society of Alexander
Technique Teachers (ISATT)
www.isatt.ie
www.stat.org.uk

ISRAEL
The Israeli Society of Teachers of the
Alexander Technique
www.alexander.org.il

NETHERLANDS
Nederlandse Vereniging van Leraren in
de Alexander Techniek (NeVLAT)
www.alexandertechniek.nl

NEW ZEALAND
Alexander Technique Teachers' Society
of New Zealand (ATTSNZ)
www.alexandertechnique.org.nz

NORWAY
Norsk Forening for Laerere i
Alexanderteknikk (NFLAT)
www.alexanderteknikk.no

SOUTH AFRICA
South African Society of Teachers of the
Alexander Technique (SASTAT)
www.alexandertechnique.org.za

SPAIN
Spanish Society of Teachers of the
Alexander Technique (APTAE)
www.aptae.net

SWITZERLAND
Schweizerischer Verband der
Lehrerinnen und Lehrer der F.M.
Alexander-Technik (SVLAT/ASPTA)
www.alexandertechnik.ch

USA
American Society for the Alexander
Technique (AmSAT)
www.alexandertech.org

Other interesting websites include:
www.alexandertechnique.org/
www.alexandertechnique.com
www.ati-net.com
www.atcongress.com
www.alexandertechniqueworldwide.com
www.mouritz.co.uk
www.mtpress.com
www.alexanderbooks.co.uk
www.bodymap.org
www.posturepage.com
www.davidreedmedia.co.uk

Further Reading

Easy-to-follow and informative books on the Alexander Technique

Brennan, Richard, *The Alexander Technique Manual*, Little Brown, 1996
Brennan, Richard, *The Alexander Technique Workbook*, Anova, 2011
Brennan, Richard, *The Alexander Technique – New Perspectives*, Chrysalis Books, 2001
Brennan, Richard, *Mind and Body Stress Relief with the Alexander Technique*, Thorsons, 1996
Chance, Jeremy, *The Alexander Technique*, Thorsons, 1998
Gelb, Michael, *Body Learning*, Aurum Press, 1981
Nicholls, Carolyn, *Body, Breath and Being*, D & B Publishing, 2008
Park, Glen, *The Art of Changing*, Ashgrove Press, 1989
Stevens, Chris, *The Alexander Technique*, Optima, 1987

More in-depth or specialized books on the Alexander Technique
Barlow, Marjorie, *An Examined Life*, Mornum Time Press, 2002
Barlow, Wilfred, *The Alexander Principle*, Gollancz, 1973
Carrington, Walter *Thinking Aloud*, Mornum Time Press, 1994
Conable, Barbara and William, *How to Learn the Alexander Technique*, Andover Press, 1991
Heirich, Jane, *Voice and the Alexander Technique*, Mornum Time Press, 2004
Macdonald, Patrick, *The Alexander Technique as I See It*, Sussex Academic Press, 1989

Maisel, Edward, *The Resurrection of the Body*, Shambala, 1969
Pierce Jones, Frank, *Body Awareness in Action / The Freedom to Change*, Shocken Books, 1976
Vineyard, Missy, *How You Stand, How You Move, How You Live*, Morlowe and Company, 2007
Westfeldt, Lulie, *F Matthias Alexander: The Man and his Work*, Centerline Press, 1964

Books by F M Alexander
The Use of the Self, Gollancz, 1985
The Universal Constant in Living, Centerline Press, 1986
Man's Supreme Inheritance, Centerline Press, 1988
Constructive Conscious Control of the Individual, Gollancz, 1987

Other related books
Bacci, Ingrid, *The Art of Effortless Living*, Perigee Books, 2002
Bacci, Ingrid, *Effortless Pain Relief*, Simon & Schuster, 2005
Doidge, Norman, *The Brain that Changes Itself*, Penguin Books, 2007
Herrigel, Eugen, *Zen in the Art of Archery*, Arkana, 1953
Liedloff, Jean, *The Continuum Concept*, Penguin Books, 1975
Tolle, Eckhart, *A New Earth*, Penguin Books, 2005

Index

Page numbers in **bold** indicate illustrations

A

acrobats 115, **116**
active lying down *see* semi-supine position
actors 16–17, 20–1, 29, 158, 164
adrenalin 79
Africa 128
Alexander, Albert Redden 29
Alexander, Frederick Matthias 10, 47, 80, 81, 109, 115, 122, 129, 131, 133–4, 135, 147, 164
 acting career 20–1
 'breathing man' 158
 case study example 31–3
 development of the Technique 29–35
 early years 19–20
 happiness 18
 influential pupils 11–12, 33–5, 104
 origins of the Technique 19–28
 and 'posture' terminology 8, 58
 quoted 37, 50, 53, 60–1, 64, 71, 77, 100, 101, 150–1, 163, 169, 170–1
 views on education 70–5
 voice problems 20–8, 36, 158
Alexander 'experience' 4–5, 149–51
Alexander lessons 47–50, **48**, **49**, 148–9
 children 36, **94**
angina 11
anxiety 78, 160
Aristotle 102, 170
arm-body joint 109–12, **111**
arthritis 42, 43, 137
asthma 43, 158, 161
atlanto-occipital joint 109, **110**
awareness 27, 47, **48**, 50, 114, 147
 of breathing 164
 exercises 131–3
Awareness (de Mello) 17

B

BackCare 43
back pain 127
 alternative treatments 45–7
 author's story 43–7
 caused by self 5, 22
 helped by semi-supine position 154–5
 and incorrect bending 112
 medical treatments 44–5
 musicians 14
 prevalence in industrialized countries 43, 54
 randomized controlled trials of treatments 177–8
 and school furniture 92

 and sitting on chairs 85
Bakewell, Joan 90
balance 39, 104, **107**, 109, 115–30, **116**, 158
 and hammer throwing 14
 and postural reflexes 58, 59
 and the senses 102
Barlow, Dr Wilfred 32, 161
Barlow, Marjorie 5, 18
'Being' 151, 175–6
being present 17–18, 39, 83, 171–4, 176, 179
bending down **41**, 106, 112–14, 124–8, **126**, **127**
body
 instability 117
 as whole unit 26, 28
 see also psycho-physical unity
body mapping 108–14
brain
 'competitive plasticity' 71–2
 and learning/unlearning 82
 and the senses 102, 104
breathing 39, 157–67
 Alexander's problems 23, 24, 28
 enjoyment of 167
 exercises 161
 how it works 162–3
 improving 156, 163–6
 performers 17
 and posture 158
 and stress 160, 164
Brennan, Tim 144–5
British Medical Journal 34–5
Bronowski, Jacob 81
Burke, Edmund 100–1
Buzan, Tony 82

C

car seats 86, 93
chairs 85–95
 backward-sloping seats **87**, 88, **89**, **91**, 92, 93–5
 cycle of discomfort 93
 height 95
 school 87–93
 tilting 88, **89**
Chappell, Greg 14, 105
children
 Alexander lessons 36, **94**
 being present 18, 76–7, 171
 bending down **41**, 106
 and education 64–75
 natural breathing 160
 natural grace 7, **15**, 39
 natural movements 57

natural standing **55**, 121
orthotics 138
posture training 56
and school chairs 87–93, **89, 91**
and school desks **69**, 95, **96, 97**
'somebody training' 172–3
time spent sitting on chairs 86–7
Christie, Linford 14
Churchill, Winston 137
Cleese, John 4, 51
Coghill, George E 16
Cole, Kelly 134
Conable, Barbara 108
Conable, William 108
conscious control 61, 170, 179
coordination 39, 58, 104, 115, 158
Cranz, Galen 85
Cripps, Stafford 35, 148

D
Dahl, Roald 4, 176
depression 18, 54, 63
Descartes, René 63
desks 95–7, **98, 99**
and bad posture in teenagers **72, 74**
school **69**, 95, **96, 97**
Dewey, John 33, 71
diaphragm 162
directions 27–8, 131, 133–7, 179
secondary 137
in semi-supine position 154
Doidge, Norman 71–2, 82
driving 7, 10, 12, 150
car seats 86, 93
posture 43, 46
Dunphy, Eamon 171

E
education 33, 64–75
Einstein, Albert 115, 117, 146
Emerson, Ralph Waldo 76
emotional habits 46–7, 51
emotions 17
in balance 115–16
and posture 169–71
and time pressure 79
see also psycho-physical unity
end-gaining *see* goal orientation
Eyeless in Gaza (Huxley) 35
eyes 120–1

F
faulty sensory appreciation 25–6, 42, 100–2,
104–8, 150–1, 166, 179
fear reflexes 12, 71, 75, 129, 179
feet
structure and design 139–41, **140**
prevalence of problems 66, 145
free choice 27, 167, 179
lacking in education 67–70
Freud, Sigmund 81
furniture 85–99

G
Gatto, John Taylor 73
Gelb, Michael 68
Gentempo, Patrick 29
Glasser, Ronald J 147
goal orientation (end-gaining) 27, 28, 77, 179
in education 75
goal-oriented exercise **106**
gravity 54, 58, 59, 115, 154

H
habits/behaviour patterns 26, 28, 37–42, 179
and brain plasticity 71–2
changing 7–8, 27, 51, 80
and fear of learning 71
formation in childhood 73–5
mental and emotional 46–7, 51
postural 37, 47, 57–8, 170
rushing 78–80
unconscious nature of 5–7, 23, 28
happiness 18, 39, 46, 50
and balance 116–17
and stressful education 69–70
and time-related stress 79–80
head
balance on the spine 117–19, **118**
directing forward and upward 136
and Primary Control 24
pulling back 23, 24, 25–6, 27, 36, 77–8,
153, 166
headaches 7, 43
head-spine (neck joint) 109, **110**
health
and posture 8–10, 53–4
preserving into old age 10–12
and stress 12
Health and Safety Executive, UK 43
heart problems 12, 78
heels (on shoes) 141–2
hip joint 112, **113**
Hippocrates 63
Hunt, Andy 145
Hurt, William 158
Huxley, Aldous 35, 79
hypertension 12, 78

I
industrialized countries 54, 57, 145
prevalence of back pain 43, 54
inhibition 27, 28, 80–2, 131, 170, 179
injuries, sports 13, 14
insomnia 35, 151
Ireland 78
ironing **38**

J
Julian, Jeff 14

K
kinaesthetic sense 102, 179
Kline, Kevin 155

L
Langford, Elizabeth 92–3
Langham, Michael 73
larynx 167
  depression 23, 24, 25
Leeper, Alexander 70
Liedloff, Jean 77
lifting 106
lightness 37–9, 149–50
'Little School, The', London 70–1
lumbar supports 112–14
lungs 162, **163**, 167
Lyons, Colette 144
Lytton, Lord 35

M
Macdonald, Peter 33–4
McCowen, Alec 119
McEnroe, John 14
McKay, Dr J W Stewart 30
Maddams, Patrick 134
means whereby 170
Merton, Thomas 116–17
mind
  in balance 116
  mental habits 46–7, 51
  and posture 18
  and time pressure 78–9
  see also psycho-physical unity
mind-body division 63
mindfulness 17–18
mind-wandering 17, 39, 171, 179
Montessori, Maria 70
Morgan, Louise 31, 33
muscles 132
  paired contraction/lengthening 61
  postural and phasic 59–61
muscular tension see tension
musculoskeletal problems 7, 60
musicians 14–16, **15**, 108, 164

N
National Back Pain Association, UK 92
National Center for Health Statistics, US 43
neck
  freeing **49**, 135–6
  head-spine joint 109, **110**, 119
neck problems 54, 127
  caused by self 5–7, 22
  musicians 14
  and reading with bifocals 121
  and school furniture 92
  and sitting on chairs 85
neuroscience 63, 71–2, 82, 134
New Earth, A (Tolle) 175

O
O'Connor, Martin 3
older people 10–12, 50
orthotics (shoe inserts) 138, 141, 145

P
phasic muscles 59–61
pain 5–8, 11, 42, 58
  as body's warning system 5, 42, 46
  see also back pain, neck problems
painkilling drugs 42, 44
Papini, Giovanni 167
Payne, Howard 14
Peanuts 8
Pearce, James 20
pelvis 92, **113**
performance enhancement 13–17
personal development 17
philosophy for living 174–6
physiotherapy 44–5
Pierce Jones, Frank 67, 81
plantar flexion reflex 143
postural habits 37, 47, 57–8, 170
postural muscles 59–61
postural reflexes 39, 58, 59, 143
posture (use) 179
  accommodation to bad (misuse) 39–42
  and breathing 158
  children 39
  'correct' 37, 53, 61
  defining 56–8
  deterioration throughout childhood 64–7
  driving 43, 46
  effects of furniture 85–99
  and emotions 169–71
  and functions 25, 28
  getting used to new 150
  and health 8–10, 53–4
  improving 8–10
  and the interoceptive senses 104
  and pain 5–7, 42
  pre-industrial people 39
  redefining 58–9
  and shoes 138–46
  and sport 14
  and stress 12
  and time pressure 76, 77–8
  and the voice 16, 24–5, 36, 166–7
  and the whole being 8, 18, 61–3,
    168–76
posture training 44, 54–6
Power of New, The (Tolle) 17
pre-industrial people 39, 43, 114
Primary Control 24, 28, 30, 109, 117–19,
  135–6, 141, 179
prolapsed discs 44
proprioception 102, 104, 133
Proust, Marcel 131
psycho-physical unity 8, 17, 22, 28, 37, 39,
  61–3, **62**, 179
public speakers 16–17, 164
pushchairs 93

R
Ram Dass (Dr Richard Alpert) 78, 171–2
reading **120**, 121
Redgrave, Lynn 142

re-education (unlearning) 50–1, 37, 52, 71–2, 82, 151
  breathing 161, 164
reflexes *see* fear reflexes; postural reflexes
Reilly, Danny 4, 45
Repetitive Strain Injury (RSI) 14
Research Board for the Correlation of Medical Science and Physical Education 66
Robbins, Anthony 81
Rolf, Ida 53
Rossi, William A 138–9, 141
Rumi 168
running, natural 143–4
rushing, habit of 78–80

S
school *see* chairs; desks; education
sciatic pain 44
Self 179
self-esteem 46, 54, 75, 174, 175
semi-supine position 151–6
senses 102–8, 174
Shaw, George Bernard 11–12, 36
Sherrington, Sir Charles 10, 35, 104
shoes 138–46
shoulders
  'pulling back' 44, 54, 59–60, 61, 121
  rounded 61, 63, 137
sitting 124
  balanced **125**
  causing strain **9**, 45–6, **125**
  at desks 95–7, **96**, **98**, **98**, **99**
  for relaxation 124
  moving to, from standing 129–30
  moving to standing 128–9
  while in activity 124
  see also chairs
'sitting bones' (ischial tuberosities) 92
'sitting up straight' 5, 53, 54–6, 59–60, 90, 158
skeleton 90–2, 109–14
soles, rigidity 142–3
'somebody training' 172–3
South American Indians 77
'speed age' 76–7
spine 112–14, 117
  alignment 151
  bending 124–6
  lengthening 136, 156
  over-curvature 11, 66, 136, 156
  pressure from school bags **65**
spirit 167
  effect of time pressure 79
sport 13–14
  winners'/losers' posture 61–3
standing 121–2
  balanced **123**
  causing strain **6**, 42, **123**
  improved 122–4
  leaning back 7, **103**
'standing up straight' 54–6, 55, 121
Stevenson, Robert Louis 168
stress 12

and breathing 160, 164
and education 68–70
and health 12
reduction, semi-supine position 151, 156
and rushing 78–80
and time pressure 12, 83–4
strokes 12, 78
surgery 44
Swift, Sally 13–14

T
Tao Te Ching 174
Tasker, Irene 70
Temple, William 35
tension 7, 39, 48, 115, 179
  awareness of 37, 52, 147, 151, 53
  awareness exercises 131–3
  and backward-sloping furniture 88
  bending down 126–7
  and breathing 158, 159, 160
  and depression 63
  and 'elderly' ailments 42
  and 'end-gaining' 27
  and faulty sensory perception 104–5
  rebalancing 37, 150
  releasing 24, 37, 50, 51, 52, 60–1, 170
  releasing through directions 135–7, 154
  sitting down 129–30
  and sports training 13
  and suppressed emotions 169–70
  and time pressure 12, 76, 80
  and the voice 166–7
Thich Nhat Hanh 157, 167
thinking in activity 179
Thompson, Daley 14
time pressure 76–84
  and breathing 157, 160
  in education 75
  and stress 12, 83–4
Tinbergen, Nikolaas 19
Twain, Mark 17

V
Vivobarefoot Shoe 145–6
voice 166–7
  Alexander's problems 20–8, 36, 158

W
Walker, Elizabeth 10
walking
  effect of shoes 138–43, 144
  natural 143
wedge-shaped cushions **91**, 93–5, **97**, **99**
'whispered ah' 164–6
Wohl, Miriam 61
Woodward, Joanne 57
writing platforms 95–6

Y
Yue, Guang 134

Z
Zumbach the tailor 173–4